OUTDOOR LIFE

THE
EMERGENCY SURVIVAL MANUAL

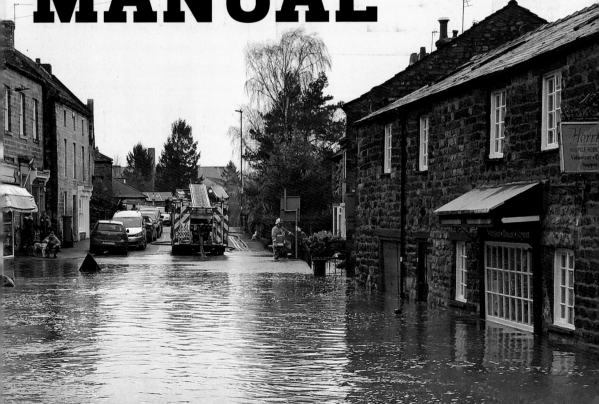

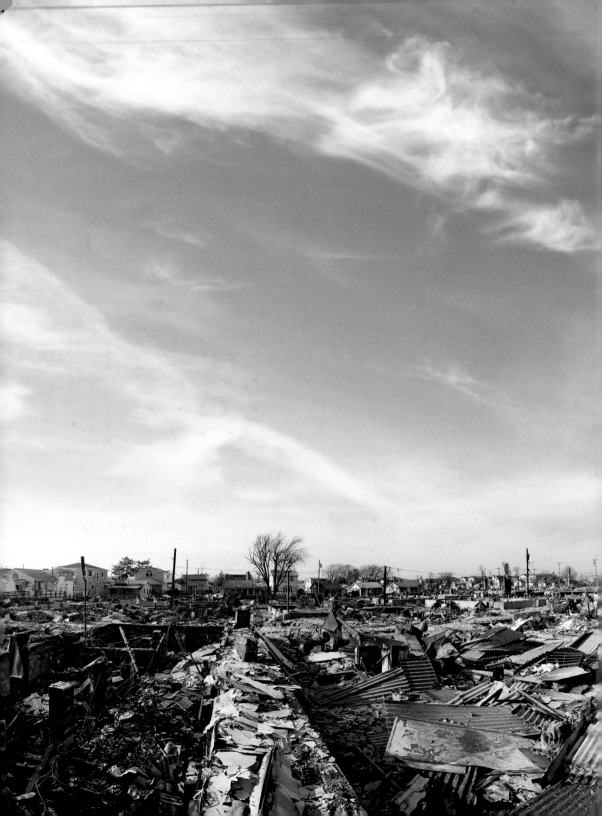

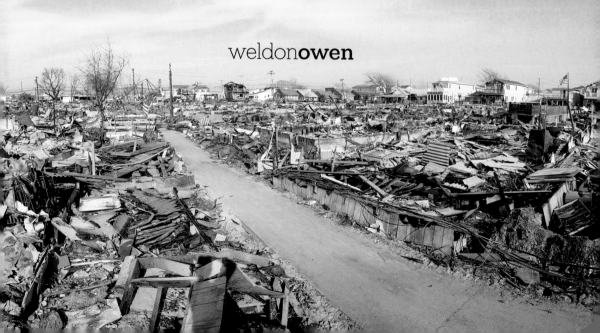

OUTDOOR LIFE

JOSEPH PRED
AND THE EDITORS OF *OUTDOOR LIFE*

THE
EMERGENCY SURVIVAL MANUAL

weldon**owen**

⬢ SKILLS

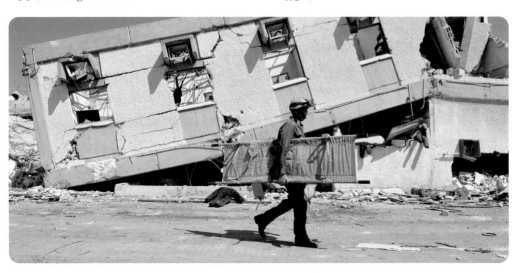

FAMILY

LIFE SAFETY APP: SOCIAL MEDIA

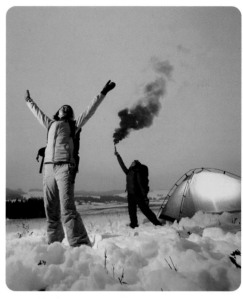

LIFE SAFETY APP: KIDS' SAFETY

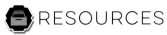

RESOURCES

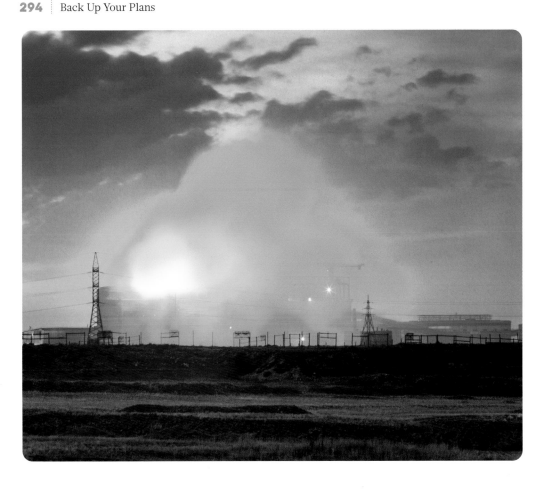

A WORST-CASE COMPANION

When we imagine ourselves in an emergency scenario, it's only natural to cast ourselves as the hero of the story. But whatever those circumstances may be, there's no way we are imagining the situation to be a fun one. When we find ourselves in a real emergency, it will truly be one of the worst days of just about anybody's entire life. It's during times like those when we will need the advice of a seasoned professional.

Non-events like Y2K and the Mayan apocalypse of 2012 gave every crackpot with a YouTube channel the opportunity to proclaim that they were a "survival expert" or "disaster specialist," regardless of their background or credibility. The coronavirus pandemic of 2020 has similarly spawned an abundance of armchair experts in all things disaster, but are those really the people you'd want to listen to when you're facing a frightening emergency on your own?

My colleague Joseph Pred has been an Emergency and Risk Manager for more than twenty years, and no one else in the survival industry—and I mean NO ONE else— can bring you the wealth of real-life disaster experience that he can deliver.

From disaster planning to threat mitigation, and from emergency response to recovery efforts, Joseph's heroic history of being a first responder has given him (and his lucky readers) a more valuable and applicable perspective than anyone else can offer. Joseph knows more than just the "parts and pieces" of survival.

He knows the value of planning and training, and maybe even more importantly, he knows how to explain these things in a way that makes emergency preparedness accessible to everyone.

There's a lot more to survival than beans, bullets, bunkers and huge over-compensating Rambo knives. Survival is about identifying your risks, preparing to meet them, and creating the back-up plans to protect yourself and those you care about. The content herein not only meets these needs, it exceeds them!

In short, this book is a gold mine of real-world emergency experience and it is a definitive lifesaving resource.

TIM MACWELCH
Director of Advanced Survival Training and author of
multiple *New York Times* Bestselling survival books

ARE YOU PREPARED?

Emergencies and disasters might feel like they belong in the realm of Hollywood movies, or something that happens to someone else. After all, it can be uncomfortable to think about circumstances where things might be out of your control and the outcome is uncertain. But the fact is emergencies happen to everyone. If you're lucky, the emergencies and disasters you face will be relatively minor, but sooner or later they will happen and affect your life in some way. This book isn't intended to scare you with worst-case scenarios, nor is it intended to be an extreme end-of-the-world 'prepper' manual. Instead, it's intended for everyday people who want to be more informed and prepared, no matter what life brings. Facing adversity is difficult under almost any circumstance, but being unprepared makes coping with those emergencies that much harder. Your willingness to increase your awareness, take steps to plan ahead, and accept that life sometimes means handling tough situations with as much calm determination as you can manifest, will help you be resilient and prevail.

Unfortunately, some of you may have had less than enjoyable experiences in the past with really dry and uninspiring material about safety, disasters, and preparedness. This book, however, is colorfully designed to be easy to read, with subjects broken down into bite-sized pieces that won't overwhelm you.

This book provides an introduction to a wide variety of skills and strategies that will be helpful in a wide range of circumstances. You can use it as a broad reference guide, or pick and choose just the content that feels most relevant to your needs. Either way, I hope it will inspire you to increase your level of preparedness, to better understand the potential hazards in your environment, to take a class to better your skills, and to volunteer to serve your community in a time of need.

If you're new to disaster preparedness, look at this book as a resource to help you and your family get started. Don't feel too much pressure to get it all done at once, or to master every skill. Instead, arm yourself with curiosity to learn some new skills and tools that will help you handle almost any crisis. There's a lot to learn, but every step you takes you farther away from being a victim and brings you closer to being a resilient survivor. If you already have your five- or seven-day emergency kit and are reading this to learn more, you'll hopefully find a new ways to solve a problem or techniques to improve your preparedness. Either way, you're bound to learn and expand your knowledge.

JOSEPH PRED
Author

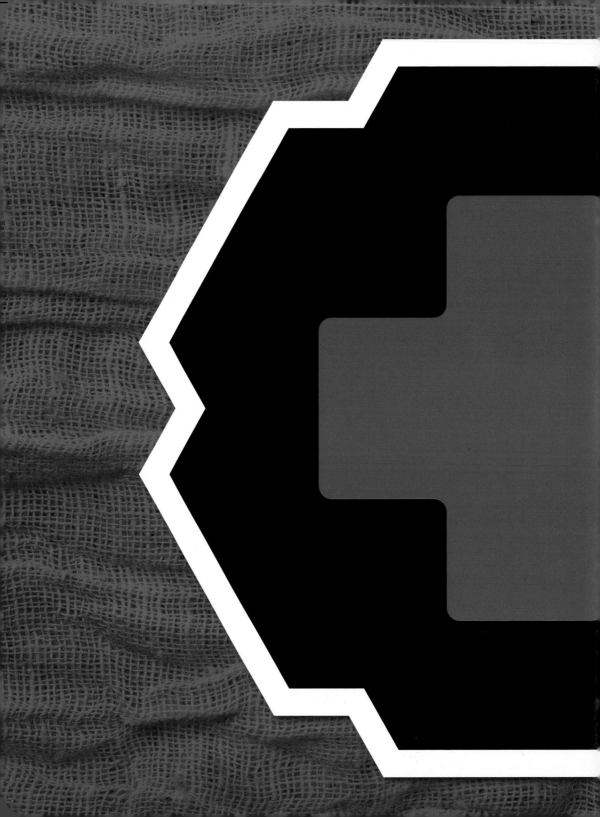

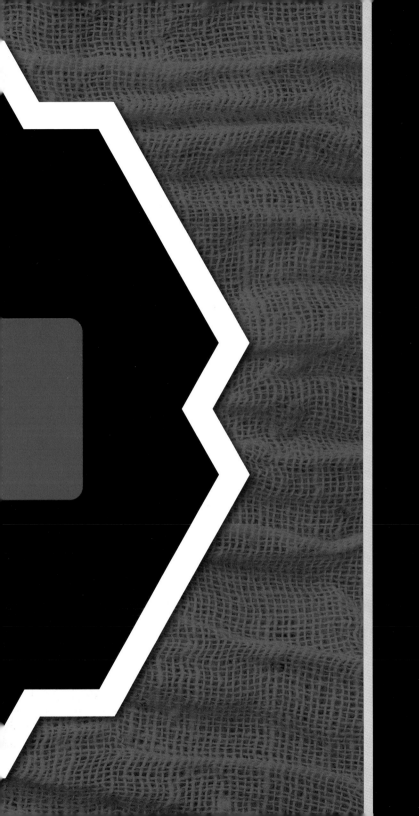

SKILLS

WHAT STARTED AS A PLEASANT CAMPING TRIP COULD HAVE EASILY TURNED TRAGIC.

A friend was petting a horse in a meadow when the horse unexpectedly kicked her in the head. She managed to stagger over to us despite bleeding from a head wound. Luckily my medical training meant that I was able to evaluate her condition (she needed stitches, but fortunately her skull wasn't fractured), and arrange to get her taken safely out of the park, and driven to a hospital for treatment. My work in public safety means that I've had many opportunities to make a difference, but this one was personal, and helping friends and family has been the most meaningful to me. I've learned that having the skills to help someone can transform a potentially scary situation into one that feels manageable.

Not knowing what to do in a difficult situation is a terrible feeling, a feeling of powerlessness. It's even worse in an emergency, when you don't have the skills to cope. We often rely on emergency responders to be there when we need them most, but in some crises you may instead have to rely on yourself and the people around you to handle the situation. The skills and gear explored in this section will help you be better prepared to handle a variety of challenging situations, from the everyday to the catastrophic. Easily stressed out or overwhelmed? You'll learn how situational awareness and crisis management techniques apply to a wide range of scenarios. Wondering about first aid? Learn how to assess shock, handle a seizure, or stop serious bleeding. Are you prepared to defend yourself? Explore different ways to fend off an attack armed with your wits or with something that has a little bit more punch. Not sure how prepared you really are? Get simple guidance on tools, medical supplies, drugs, and protective equipment so you can be ready to handle the next emergency; because having the right basic skills and tools is the first step towards to overcoming adversity.

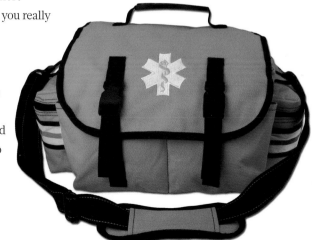

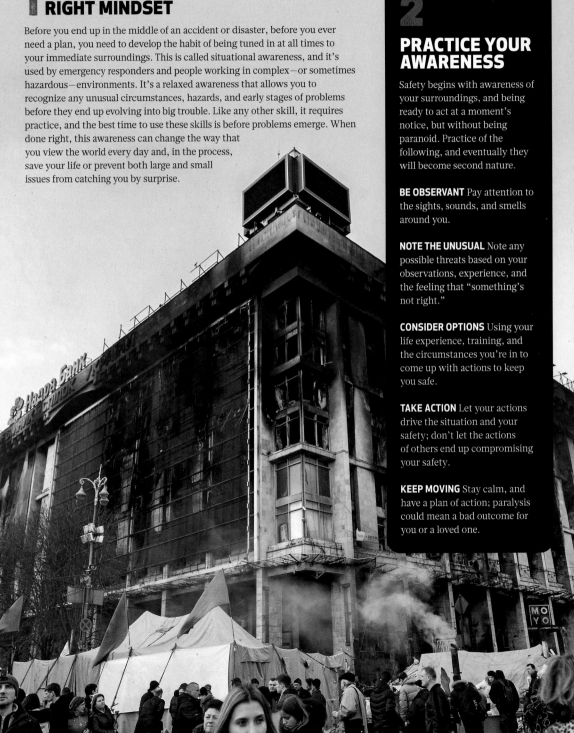

1 GET THE RIGHT MINDSET

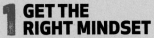

Before you end up in the middle of an accident or disaster, before you ever need a plan, you need to develop the habit of being tuned in at all times to your immediate surroundings. This is called situational awareness, and it's used by emergency responders and people working in complex—or sometimes hazardous—environments. It's a relaxed awareness that allows you to recognize any unusual circumstances, hazards, and early stages of problems before they end up evolving into big trouble. Like any other skill, it requires practice, and the best time to use these skills is before problems emerge. When done right, this awareness can change the way that you view the world every day and, in the process, save your life or prevent both large and small issues from catching you by surprise.

2

PRACTICE YOUR AWARENESS

Safety begins with awareness of your surroundings, and being ready to act at a moment's notice, but without being paranoid. Practice of the following, and eventually they will become second nature.

BE OBSERVANT Pay attention to the sights, sounds, and smells around you.

NOTE THE UNUSUAL Note any possible threats based on your observations, experience, and the feeling that "something's not right."

CONSIDER OPTIONS Using your life experience, training, and the circumstances you're in to come up with actions to keep you safe.

TAKE ACTION Let your actions drive the situation and your safety; don't let the actions of others end up compromising your safety.

KEEP MOVING Stay calm, and have a plan of action; paralysis could mean a bad outcome for you or a loved one.

3 COLOR YOUR PERCEPTIONS

To better understand situational awareness, it's useful to see it as a scale. More important, you can consciously move up or down the scale as part of stress management or checking in with yourself about how aware you are in the moment. It's a good exercise to ask yourself occasionally, "What color am I at right now?"

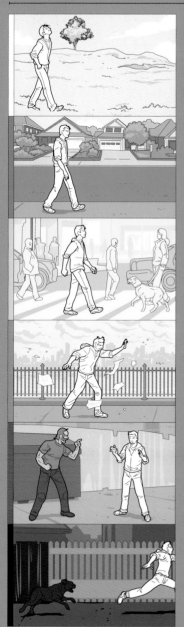

WHITE (UNAWARE) Your head is in the clouds. You are unlikely to notice if anything dangerous is unfolding around you, nor are you be prepared to react. This lack of awareness is aggravated by being distracted or emotional, or having a false sense of security. Physical issues like sleep deprivation, pain, stress, or intoxication can also dull your awareness. This white level of awareness is like being drowsy behind the wheel of your car.

GREEN (RELAXED) This low level of awareness is reserved for very safe places. You're ready to increase your awareness to Yellow if something unusual happens but isn't likely to happen. This is how you might feel relaxing at home in a safe neighborhood. Switching back to Green after coming home from dealing with an Orange or Red situation is an important part of consciously managing stress.

YELLOW (AWARE) Calm and alert, you have a relaxed awareness of your surroundings. This is how emergency responders are while on duty. At this level, you're observant of all things—aware of people, animals, environmental conditions, and the layout or terrain of an area. You can react quickly if your situation changes. This is similar to the alertness needed for normal defensive driving on a busy road.

ORANGE (POSSIBLE PROBLEM) There may be a problem; you're starting to process information that causes concern for your safety. At this level, you're noticing that something is wrong and are evaluating options for reacting to the situation. This is an ideal time to proactively move to a safer location or change what you're doing before things get ugly. Consider this level similar to that needed for driving in very bad weather or on an icy road.

RED (THREAT) You're in trouble. You have to act now for your safety or defend yourself. The time for assessing options is over. Pick your target or escape route, and move! This level is like reacting to a car pulling in front of you when you're traveling at high speed in bad weather; there's a split second to decide whether to hit the car or swerve into another lane. If you have been practicing situational awareness, you'll already know your options almost instinctively.

BLACK (OVERWHELMED) You're in panic mode, thinking too much and failing to act. Maybe you're paralyzed with fear or indecision, or exhibiting panicked or inappropriate behavior (whether or not you're aware of it). You can get into this mode when, say, you freeze behind the wheel during an accident, hit another car, and flip over. You may not even know what just happened or why you're upside down. You're lucky to be alive!

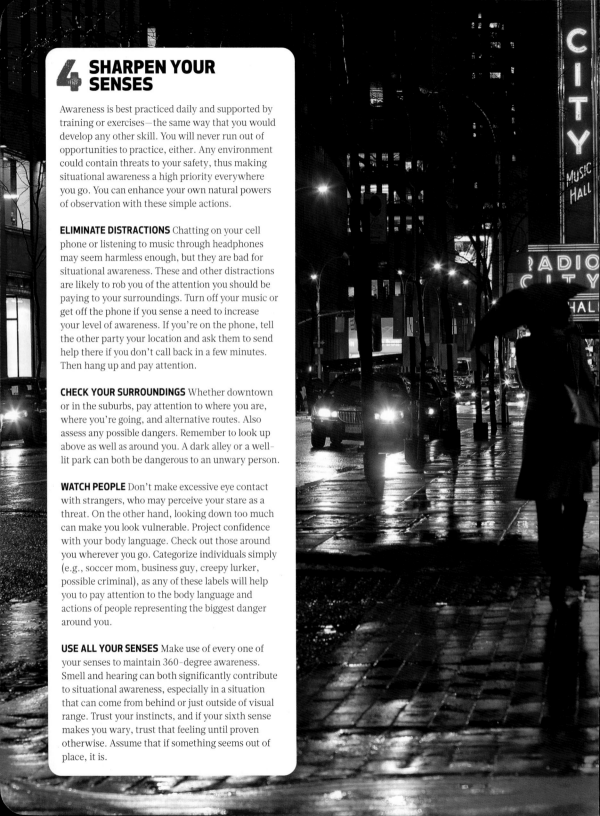

4 SHARPEN YOUR SENSES

Awareness is best practiced daily and supported by training or exercises—the same way that you would develop any other skill. You will never run out of opportunities to practice, either. Any environment could contain threats to your safety, thus making situational awareness a high priority everywhere you go. You can enhance your own natural powers of observation with these simple actions.

ELIMINATE DISTRACTIONS Chatting on your cell phone or listening to music through headphones may seem harmless enough, but they are bad for situational awareness. These and other distractions are likely to rob you of the attention you should be paying to your surroundings. Turn off your music or get off the phone if you sense a need to increase your level of awareness. If you're on the phone, tell the other party your location and ask them to send help there if you don't call back in a few minutes. Then hang up and pay attention.

CHECK YOUR SURROUNDINGS Whether downtown or in the suburbs, pay attention to where you are, where you're going, and alternative routes. Also assess any possible dangers. Remember to look up above as well as around you. A dark alley or a well-lit park can both be dangerous to an unwary person.

WATCH PEOPLE Don't make excessive eye contact with strangers, who may perceive your stare as a threat. On the other hand, looking down too much can make you look vulnerable. Project confidence with your body language. Check out those around you wherever you go. Categorize individuals simply (e.g., soccer mom, business guy, creepy lurker, possible criminal), as any of these labels will help you to pay attention to the body language and actions of people representing the biggest danger around you.

USE ALL YOUR SENSES Make use of every one of your senses to maintain 360-degree awareness. Smell and hearing can both significantly contribute to situational awareness, especially in a situation that can come from behind or just outside of visual range. Trust your instincts, and if your sixth sense makes you wary, trust that feeling until proven otherwise. Assume that if something seems out of place, it is.

5 SHAKE YOUR TAIL

Usually someone is walking behind you because they just happen to be going your way, but occasionally it may be because they want to harass you, mug you, or worse. Listen to your instincts and take action to avoid being a victim. Here are some tactics to use.

STAY COOL Don't confront the person following you. Focus instead on getting to safety.

REFLECT ON MATTERS Use windows and mirrors to look back instead of turning around or looking over your shoulder. Both of those actions can give you away.

CHANGE COURSE By changing directions, crossing the street, or making several turns, you can easily verify if you're being followed.

GET ON CAMERA Keep an eye out for CCTV security cameras and make sure to walk past them, hopefully catching the person on video in the process. Alternatively, you can put your mobile phone into video mode to capture a record of what happens. Don't point the camera at him in any obvious way; instead try to briefly bring the phone up as if you're checking it while capturing his image.

STAY SAFE Stay in well-lit areas and avoid deserted places such as alleys or empty side streets.

GO PUBLIC Board public transit such as a bus, subway, or light rail; the more crowded the better. Exit right before the doors close if the pursuer also boards.

BUY SOME TIME Enter a store, restaurant, or another public place to consider your options. You're more safe with people around. Consider buying a ticket to a movie, then leave the theater through an emergency exit before the tail enters.

GET HELP Call a friend or hail a cab to pick you up, or call the police if you feel unsafe.

CROWD SURF Walk in the middle of a large crowd, if one is available, to stay hidden from view. It's safer than going walking alone.

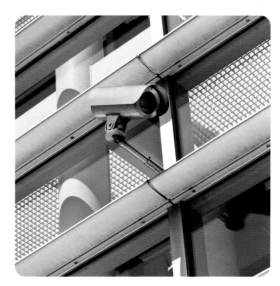

6 AVOID AUTOMATIC BEHAVIOR

You know that feeling you get when you've driven your regular commute route, or ridden the usual subway, and you realize that you're now at work without having a conscious thought as to how you got there? You have just engaged in automatic behavior! It's most easily triggered while traveling along very familiar routes. This can represent a very dangerous threat to your situational awareness. You can avoid falling into automatic behavior by consciously staying in a state of relaxed awareness. Automatic behavior is another way one is in White when they should be in Yellow (see item 3).

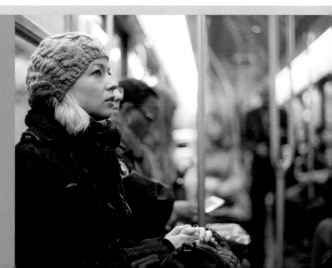

7 KEEP YOURSELF IN THE LOOP

The OODA Loop was originally created by military strategist and fighter pilot Colonel John Boyd, and has since become a useful tool in environments including survival, litigation, sports, politics, and business. It's versatile enough to apply to all sorts of planning, and it can provide a streamlined framework to organize responses in reactive circumstances.

The OODA Loop will help you to thrive in circumstances that are uncertain and evolving. It can be applied to both personal defense and disasters—in fact, it's useful in just about any situation. Practicing also allows you to move through the decision loop quickly and effectively; a faster understanding of the circumstances will give you a greater edge over your opponent or environment.

As you go through the loop, you must remain willing to restart to react to changing circumstances. In a highly dynamic situation the need to reorient can happen almost continuously. After all, there's no point in executing a plan after circumstances have changed and thus rendered that plan irrelevant.

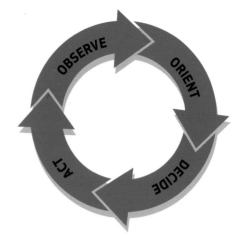

OBSERVE Using your situational awareness, gather as much information from your senses and other sources as possible. Assess if any forces in the situation will directly, indirectly, or passively affect you.

ORIENT Analyze your situation while remaining aware of your biases, past experiences, and cultural norms. Use this information to update your perspective on the situation. As new information develops you will need to integrate it quickly to revise your orientation.

DECIDE Decisions in changing circumstances are not fixed; they are fluid and must be reassessed as the loop cycles, prompted by any changes during the observation and orientation stages.

ACT Follow through on your decision, and then immediately return to the Observe stage as you evaluate the effects of your actions.

8 PERFECT AWARENESS THROUGH PRACTICE

While you are walking, driving, or engaging in everyday activity by yourself, try practicing your situational awareness by choosing to dial it up or down consciously. Some find it helpful to say observations out loud or to work together with a friend or family member to "double up" on the eyes and ears of your situational awareness. Or have them randomly ask you questions about your surroundings to make sure you're actually aware of notable issues. Another technique is to have them ask you for an escape route or what you would choose to do if a specific problem emerged. This sort of regular virtual training for situations that are unpredictable, and thus less accessible to prepare for, has shown to improve decision making when the real thing goes down.

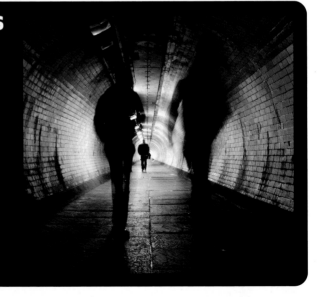

9 ADAPT AND OVERCOME

There is a well-known saying, courtesy of Prussian Field Marshal Helmuth von Moltke: "No plan survives contact with the enemy." It's important that, in both your planning process and in reacting to changing circumstances, you maintain a flexible mindset. The "enemy" could be severe weather, an earthquake, or a bad traffic accident—anything unpredictable that can harm you or hamper your progress. So create plans, but be open-minded in order to adjust to the changing circumstances. If you are rigid in your approach, your outcomes will be more limited.

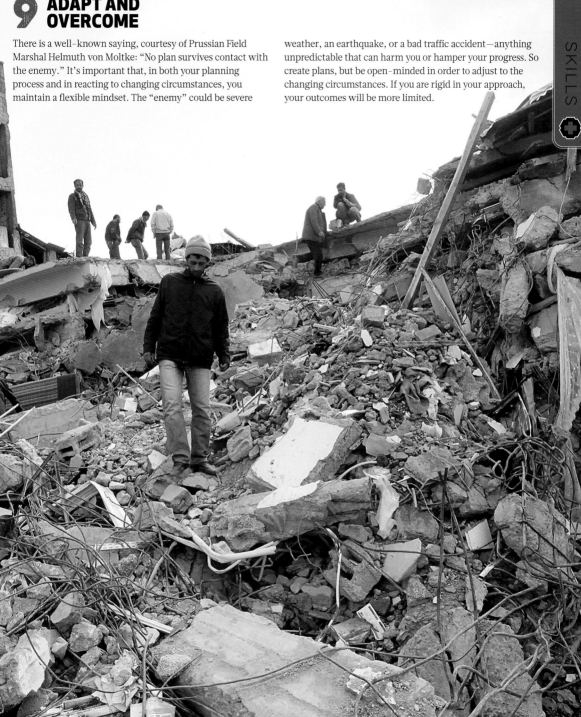

10 CALL EMERGENCY SERVICES

Regardless of where you live, there are emergency numbers available for you to use. Most countries now have a three-digit number for emergency medical services, but there is often more than one number. Some dial directly to a specific agency; there are others for local, state, and national services.

Before traveling to a new place, look up at least the local three-digit emergency number and program it into your mobile phone. If your local emergency number is 911, and you're traveling to Sweden (where the number is 112 instead) consider programming your phone with it listed as "911 Sweden," as it's common to think of your home emergency number first in a high-stress situation. Alternatively, there are smartphone apps with emergency numbers programmed for many countries—great for those who travel frequently.

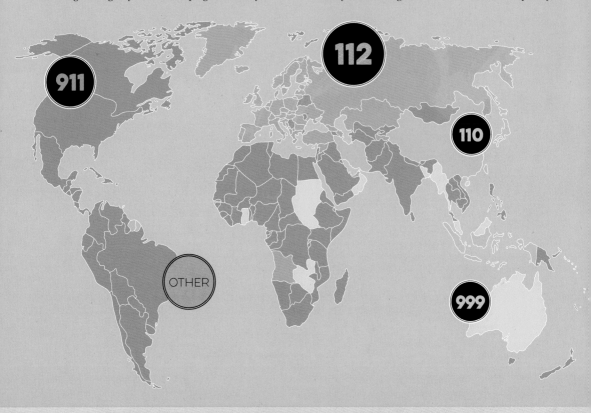

11 DIAL DIRECT

It's a lesser-known fact that you can dial to various emergency agencies directly rather than using the three-digit number. It can be worthwhile to look up your local police, fire, and other emergency medical services and add them into your phone. In some areas dialing the three-digit number on your cell phone connects to a central dispatch center to route your call. This can mean additional hold time and delays in getting you the help you need.

Dialing direct skips this step and is also useful in case the three-digit number is overloaded or unavailable. If you also keep your phone programmed with the local nonemergncy numbers, you can report lesser issues without having to use the emergency line.

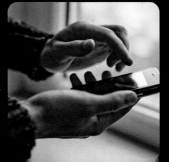

12 HANDLE IT YOURSELF

This book simultaneously addresses two different sets of circumstances for emergencies you might face: the ones that can occur during everyday unremarkable events, and those happening during large incidents or regional disasters. In both situations you'll reach a point when you'll need help and, during normal circumstances, calling local emergency services will be the easiest and best way to do so. However, during a larger incident or in a disaster, telephone lines and emergency resources may be overwhelmed. You may have to rely on the resources you have at hand to handle the situation you're facing, or transport an injured party directly to the hospital because no ambulances are available.

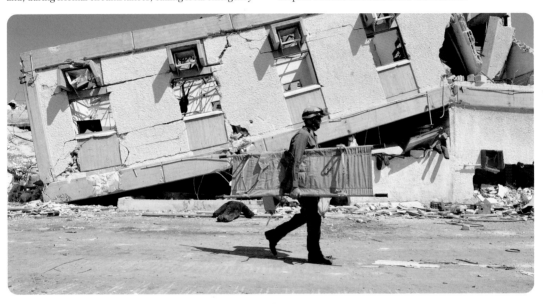

13 GET PROFESSIONAL HELP

Unless you're a trained emergency responder or medical professional, much of this section will present things you've never had to do before. Under normal circumstances, you'll hopefully never have to use them, and the instructional items in this book aren't intended to replace professional training or medical care.

In some cases, this book should only be considered a last resort, but in a disaster situation, it may very well be that you must rely on your own ingenuity and determination to survive. That said, you should always strive to get someone to proficient medical care whenever possible rather than trying something on your own. If you'd like to be better prepared, consider getting trained as a disaster volunteer to build skills and gain experience for when disaster strikes. Not only will you be able to help yourself, you'll also be a resource for your neighborhood and community.

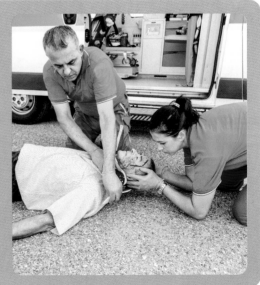

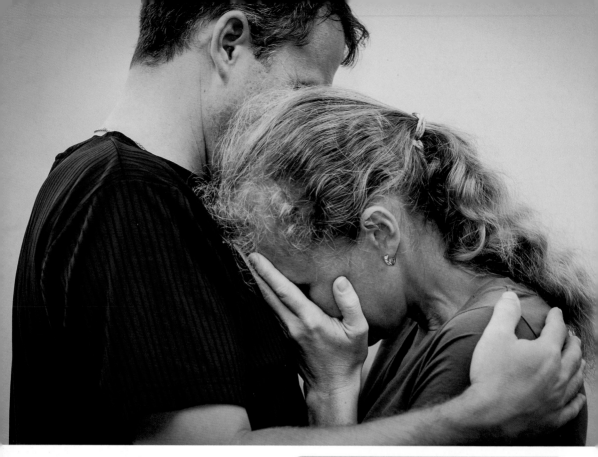

14 UNDERSTAND AND ACCEPT STRESS

Stress is a part of being human. People experience it in a variety of ways in everyday circumstances, at school, at work, and in family life. However, the type of stress you experience during an emergency or large-scale incident can be severe; understanding how it could affect you or others is an important part of self-care and helping others. Everyone who sees or experiences a disaster is affected by it in some way.

It is, for example, normal to feel anxious about your safety and that of your family and friends immediately following an incident. Other normal reactions include a deep sense of sadness, grief, or anger.

Accepting that all of these reactions and feelings are normal can help you to recover more quickly than the people who are lacking this awareness. Integrating the experience can take a long time, sometimes years, and it isn't always easy. Seek the help of mental health professionals or support groups if you feel as if you can't cope on your own.

15 RECOGNIZE SIGNS OF STRESS

People handle stress in many different ways. Even with support and resources, some individuals find themselves unable to cope. Knowing the signs of overwhelming stress can help you decide when to get assistance.

People under significant stress can experience physical reactions including fatigue, unexpected or prolonged cold- or flu-like symptoms, tunnel vision or muffled hearing, headache or stomach problems, or loss of appetite. They may report feeling confused or overwhelmed, with trouble communicating or paying attention. Their emotions may range from sadness, guilt, or frustration to fear, anger, outright denial, or emotional detachment. Conversely, they might also exhibit hyperactivity or hypervigilance, have nightmares or trouble sleeping, wild mood swings, or emotional outbursts. They may feel isolated, afraid of crowds or of being alone.

If you observe someone exhibiting these signs, they may need crisis counseling or stress management support.

TEND TO VICARIOUS TRAUMA

Indirect stress, sometimes referred to as secondary or vicarious stress, is sometimes overlooked when considering who is in need of help after a disaster. Vicarious stress can affect anyone: professional emergency responders or disaster volunteers, family members who support relatives and their communities cope with the aftermath, even those who watch too much news coverage of an incident. This secondary stress is experienced is very real, and it manifests in much the same way as those who directly experienced the event. You can use the same stress-management strategies for those who are direct victims of a disaster, and to help others who may not realize they are affected, since they "weren't there" when the incident in question happened.

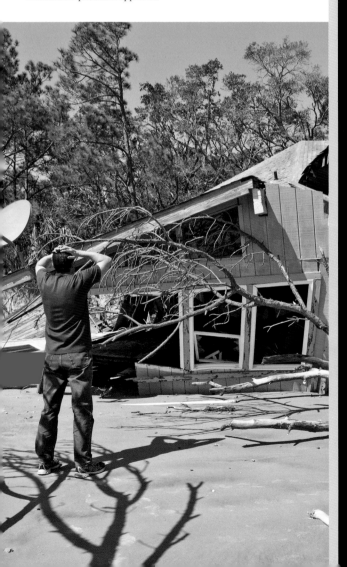

17 MANAGE YOUR MENTAL HEALTH

There are many healthy ways to manage and cope with stress, and to support others in their stress management. You know what's best for you in general, but consider accepting the help offered by community programs and resources to make your recovery easier. Your existing support network of family, friends, and any religious institutions may be also affected if the disaster is community wide, so get a mix of support from people who are not directly affected as well as from those who can relate because they've shared similar experiences. Recognize that you need to care for your physical, emotional, psychological and spiritual needs.

TEND TO YOUR BODY Get enough sleep and exercise, and eat a balanced diet. Establish a moderate balance between work, pleasure, and downtime.

CONNECT WITH OTHERS Spend time with family and friends. Be open to receiving as well as giving support. As soon as possible after the incident, reestablish your normal family or daily routine while limiting any demanding responsibilities on yourself and your family.

KEEP YOUR SPIRITS UP Use spiritual resources you have available, and be willing to talk to mental health professionals. Or just talk with someone about your feelings even though it may be difficult. It's important, however, not to force yourself or others to do so.

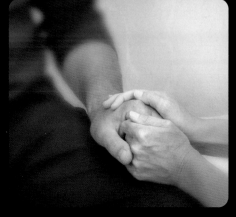

18 SUIT UP FOR SAFETY

It's counterintuitive, but personal protective equipment (PPE) is not a good source of safety—it's actually considered your last line of defense under normal circumstances. In traditional risk management, the best way to handle any risk is to eliminate it entirely, or replace it with a safer option before you have to engage with it. Administrative controls can also be used to raise awareness through the use of signs and safety monitors.

However, in a disaster situation, personal protective equipment may be your only line of defense, which is why it's so important to have access to PPE. It's also important to assign somebody to take the role of safety monitor, in order to help to maintain safety in circumstances where better options do not exist.

19 MASK UP

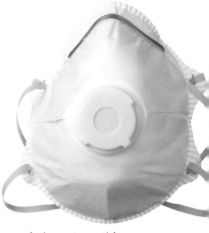

Disasters (and everyday projects) frequently involve exposure to harmful chemicals and toxins, but a mask goes far in protecting your lungs and health. Respirators and dust masks come in a variety of types and ratings. Particulate filters, including dust masks, are disposable or have replacement filters. They protect from airborne particles—including dust, mists, liquids, and some fumes—but not gases or vapors. Not all are created equal, so be sure your mask is the right one for the task.

Particulate filters are rated by the National Institute of Occupational Safety and Health (NIOSH), according to their capacity. The ratings have both a letter and number: N (not oil-proof), R (oil-resistant up to 8 hours), and P (oil-proof beyond 8 hours). Particulate filters are rated 95, 97, or 100, corresponding to the percentage of micrometer particles removed. Filters rated 100 are considered high-efficiency (HE or HEPA) filters.

The most common rating for a disposable dust mask is N95, which filters 95 percent of non-oil-based airborne particles. N95 covers basic but essential safety needs such as mold, allergens, or airborne diseases. If you need the highest level of protection in the widest variety of situations, go for P100.

20 WEAR IT PROPERLY

For the best fit and safety, there are a few useful tips to follow when wearing protective masks.

Durable half or full masks provide a better fit and protection, but disposable masks will be easier to find, however they won't seal as well. Disposable masks with an exhalation valve will make breathing easier. For higher-risk environments, choose a full face mask and disinfect after each use. Masks with an exhalation valve may make breathing easier. For higher-risk environments (such as asbestos), choose a non-disposable mask with sealing gaskets.

21 PUT THE RIGHT ONE ON

This chart will help you decide what kind of mask you should wear, depending on the substance in question.

RATING	SUBSTANCES
N95 OR HIGHER	Allergens, bacteria and viruses, bleach, dust, non-asbestos fibers, insulation, mold, pollen, debris from sanding and welding
N100 OR HEPA	Asbestos, lead
P95 OR HIGHER	Paint, pesticides, sprays

22 GET GOOD GLOVES

There is a dizzying array of glove options to keep you safe inthe field, and each type of glove protects against different hazards. Get to know the pros and cons of a few basic glove types that you're likely to consider for your PPE needs. For medical gloves [A] your best material choice is nitrile. These gloves are safe for people with latex allergies—an increasing concern in health care. For improved dexterity, stock up on textured gloves. You can also put on vinyl or polyethylene (plastic) gloves, but they are less protective. Avoid using high-priced durable gloves because, once they have been contaminated with bodily fluids, the gloves are no longer considered safe and should be discarded. For a general-purpose work glove [B], consider a modern hybrid type that may combine synthetic fibers with leather, plastic, and other materials for the best comfort, dexterity, durability, and grip. The tradeoff for this balance is that these hybrids are outdone by gloves specifically designed for just one or two factors. For example, a pair of heavy canvas or leather gloves will be more durable than hybrid work gloves. However, heavy materials need to be broken in, can be incredibly uncomfortable to wear, and may cause blisters or abrasions on your hands.Tactical gloves [C], sometimes also referred to as police gloves, are good general-purpose wear when not giving first aid or doing search-and-rescue work. They offer a variety of protection such as Kevlar linings to make them puncture- or cut-resistant while also providing excellent grip, warmth, and dexterity. Avoid riot gloves or search gloves, since the former are aggressive and can suggest to others that you're looking for a fight, while the latter offer you very little in the way of protection or warmth, since their primary function is sensitive dexterity while frisking subjects.

Ⓐ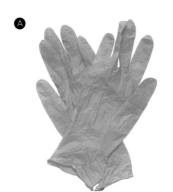

Ⓑ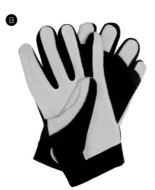

Ⓒ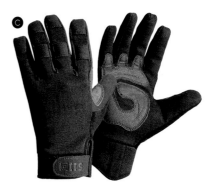

23 CHANGE GLOVES OFTEN

Any of the disposable medical gloves degrade over time, which reduces their effectiveness in protecting you from potentially contagious body fluids while rendering first aid. While standard procedure is to change gloves after every patient in medical contexts, in other situations people tend to wear the same pair of gloves for many hours at a time, but this is not recommended. Oils from your hands, skin lotion, chemicals, disinfectants, heat, and other elements all degrade the protection of your disposable gloves. When in doubt, replace your gloves!

24 DON'T BE A HERO

Equipping yourself with all of the very best of the personal protective equipment may make you feel like a superhero, but, the reality is, none of this is armor. You should still approach hazards as if you have no PPE on. This way, you're consciously avoiding any overconfidence you might gain from all the gear that you are wearing. And overconfidence can kill you as it's killed others in the past. Remember that PPE is your last resort for safety, and the best way to handle risk is to avoid it entirely whenever possible.

25 PROTECT YOURSELF

If you need to aid in a disaster or emergency incident, or if you're in an official function, you need the right gear for the job. Here's a list of what you'll need to wear to have a full suite of personal protective equipment.

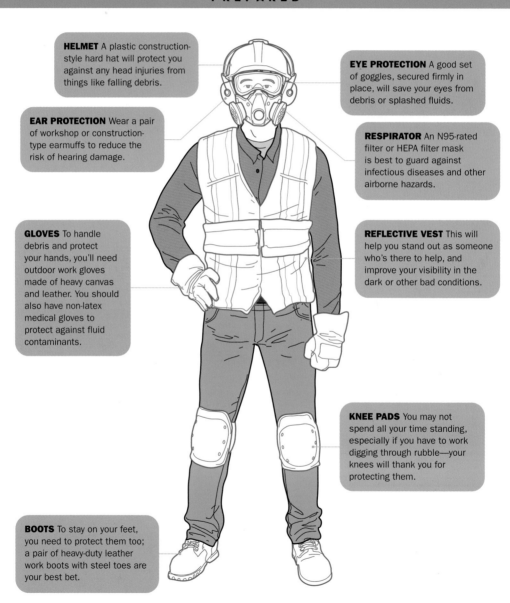

HELMET A plastic construction-style hard hat will protect you against any head injuries from things like falling debris.

EAR PROTECTION Wear a pair of workshop or construction-type earmuffs to reduce the risk of hearing damage.

GLOVES To handle debris and protect your hands, you'll need outdoor work gloves made of heavy canvas and leather. You should also have non-latex medical gloves to protect against fluid contaminants.

EYE PROTECTION A good set of goggles, secured firmly in place, will save your eyes from debris or splashed fluids.

RESPIRATOR An N95-rated filter or HEPA filter mask is best to guard against infectious diseases and other airborne hazards.

REFLECTIVE VEST This will help you stand out as someone who's there to help, and improve your visibility in the dark or other bad conditions.

KNEE PADS You may not spend all your time standing, especially if you have to work digging through rubble—your knees will thank you for protecting them.

BOOTS To stay on your feet, you need to protect them too; a pair of heavy-duty leather work boots with steel toes are your best bet.

There may be a situation for which you haven't been properly trained, or, for whatever reason, you don't have the right equipment with you. If you have to improvise your own PPE, here's how to keep yourself safer than nothing.

IMPROVISED

EYE PROTECTION Goggles are ideal, but if nothing else, a pair of sunglasses or regular glasses will help shield your eyes.

RESPIRATOR A painter's dust mask or bandanna offers little protection, especially against infectious substances, but it's better than nothing.

VEST If you don't have a reflective vest, look for something else bright that stands out well, like a neon-colored or tie-dyed shirt.

BOOTS Rain boots or hiking boots are not as sturdy as work boots or similar footwear; nonetheless, they'll cover your feet better than flip-flops or sneakers.

HELMET Any head protection is better than none at all; for example, a bicycle helmet, which is already made to guard against head impacts, may be adequate.

EAR PROTECTION Disposable foam earplugs will protect your hearing, though keeping them clean and trying not to lose them when you remove them briefly is a hassle.

GLOVES A set of gardening gloves and/or a pair of rubber kitchen or cleaning gloves will help to keep your hands safe.

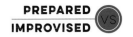

26 GET IT ON TAPE

There are lots of different types of tapes available, but not all are created equal.
Get familiar with them so you can use the right tool for the right job.

1 STICK WITH THE STANDARD Duct tape, that venerable staple, derives its toughness from a composite of woven cotton cloth that's been backed with polyethylene and then coated with a high-tack adhesive. This tape can create a waterproof seal, which makes it perfect for everything from HVAC installations to impromptu repairs to almost anything.

2 PRACTICE MEDICINE Medical tape comes in a variety of types, so it's important to know which are the best for general use. The best tape for general field use is Durapore or Curasilk. Both are strong cloth tapes with good adhesion and a smooth outside texture that doesn't catch on clothing during movement. They can be used to secure dressings, or for immobilization, and for nonmedical purposes too.

3 GET INTO SPORTS Not to be confused with medical tape, sports tape is great for reinforcing muscles and bones during rigorous physical activity of any kind, whether you're running for fun or for your life. It can also be used for anatomical tape splints to help reduce swelling, restrict movement to promote healing, and protect from reinjury.

4 CLOSE WOUNDS Steri-Strips, a special type of wound-closure tape, are the bigger, stronger cousin of the butterfly bandage. Commonly combined with tincture of benzoin for a better bond, they're used after surgery and as a substitute for stitches. Steri-Strips should only be placed on cleaned wounds with no ragged edges. Avoid using paper tape or transparent medical tape; these are not waterproof and don't work well outside a hospital setting.

5 BE AN ELECTRICIAN Besides the obvious use, electrical tape can be used to mark equipment and, as it comes in a rainbow of colors, is great for color-coding equipment, cords, and connectors. Made of slightly stretchy PVC vinyl, and backed with a pressure sensitive rubber-type adhesive, it peels off easily and usually without residue.

6 REFLECT ON IT Reflective tape comes in a variety of colors and patterns. It can mark equipment, object edges, doorways, openings, and vehicles—really almost anything that you want to be able to clearly mark for high-visibility daytime and nighttime safety.

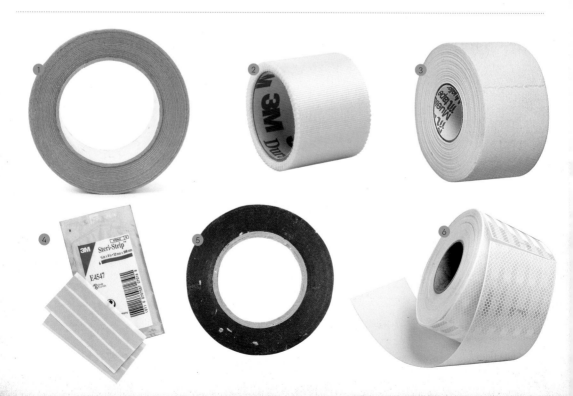

27 TOOL UP WITH TAPE

Aside from sticking two things together, duct tape can be turned to plenty of other uses. A few obvious ones include sealing cracks—whether found in plastic bottles or glass windows—or patching torn clothing or tents, but the possibilities are nearly endless. If you are using duct tape to fix a broken water bottle or hydration bladder, be sure the surface is thoroughly dry before you apply the tape.

If you're in need of a light rope or cordage, twist one or more strips together to cover the adhesive side of the tape and form a tight strand. Knots tied in a regular rope can also be reinforced and kept from slipping by simply winding a bit of duct tape around them.

The sticky stuff is also a great insulator. You can line a jacket with strips of duct tape to keep heat in, or cover the surface to keep rain out.

Duct tape can be used to not only seal containers but make them as well. For example, you can create a bowl or cup by placing several strips over your knee or a similarly rounded object, and then reinforcing both sides of the shape you have created with more tape.

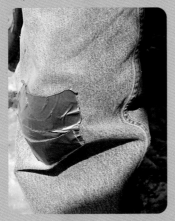

While many other forms of adhesive tape have unique, specialized purposes, none can beat duct tape in its versatility, so keep at least one roll of this stuff inside your toolbox or emergency kit.

28 BE A DUCT TAPE DOCTOR

Duct tape is highly useful for putting all sorts of things together—and that also includes the human body. This versatile material can be employed in your medical kit; here are just a few of a multitude of ways.

BANDAGE WOUNDS If you're out of proper bandages, apply gauze or other sterile dressing to a wound, then carefully hold in place with an appropriately sized strip of duct tape.

REPLACE TWEEZERS Need to remove a splinter or other object in the skin? Apply a little patch of tape and peel or pinch to remove it.

SPLINT A LIMB Use other stabilizing items such as folded cardboard or a pair of sticks to hold the injured limb steady, then wrap with a few strips of duct tape to hold in place.

FASHION A SLING Lay out a triangle of duct tape strips (with each side as long as the patient's forearm). Add a few strips inside the triangle to make a net to hold the arm. Back the strips with more tape to keep them from sticking, then secure around the arm and shoulder.

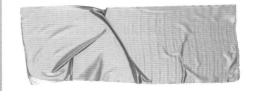

29 ESCAPE DUCT TAPE HANDCUFFS

If you've found yourself in a situation where your wrists are bound with duct tape, there's a chance you can actually escape your bonds pretty easily. Hold your hands out in front of you, bring your arms up high over your head, then, with all your strength, bring them back down fast and pull your wrists apart hard. The duct tape may well split under the force.

A note—this works only if your wrists are bound side by side, not crossed, and you will need to have your hands in front of you to make it happen. Remember those things if you need to restrain a dangerous person yourself with duct tape!

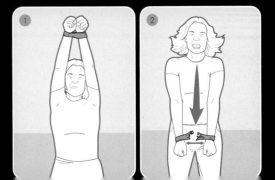

30 KEEP PARACORD HANDY

Paracord, was (as the name suggests) first used in parachutes in World War II. In the field, paratroopers discovered that this material was useful for everything from rigging tents to sawing logs. It's almost as handy as duct tape and is a virtual multitool for emergency kits.

Even better, it doesn't have to be just spooled up and stashed away. This handy material can be woven into a variety of accessories from lanyards to keychains to belts to bracelets; wound around knife, axe, or tool handles; and, of course, used to lace your boots. Thus, it can be kept right at hand for the moment when you need it. Let's take a look at some of its many versatile uses.

31 LIFT AND LOWER LOADS (NOT PEOPLE)

Paracord is also known as 550 cord because the most common variant is usually rated to hold a weight of up to 550 pounds (250 kg) before breaking, due to its construction and the several internal strands within the sheath (called the kermantle). It's a useful stand-in for rope if you need to haul something up, lower an object down (rigging cord in a pulley system to handle heavier items), or drag objects along.

A word of warning, though: If you need rope for climbing, you're better off using actual climbing rope, which is rated for a much higher weight and is made to handle active loads (such as a person bouncing around a little as they climb) and shock loading (for example, when the rope takes up the weight of a falling object) without breaking. Proper climbing rope is much thicker; paracord's versatility is partly in its size, but it's a thin cord. Trying to climb with it can lead to injury as it can be easily severed while loaded with your weight.

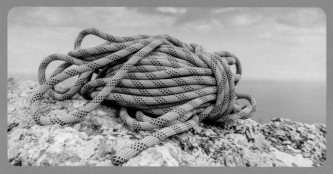

32 BECOME A STRING SURGEON

Paracord is a wonderful utility material; it also has a wide range of applications for personal and medical use.

SUTURE INJURIES Those same strands can be an emergency substitute for stitching a wound.

TOURNIQUET A LIMB To stop severe, uncontrolled bleeding, wind a few turns of paracord around the limb before twisting the cord with an inserted stick or similar to make a tourniquet (see item 82). Braiding multiple strands together will reduce the risk of limb damage.

TIE SLINGS OR SPLINTS Stabilize broken bones with cardboard, sticks, or other rigid materials, then tie them into place with paracord. You can also make a sling for an injured arm.

RESCUE A RING FINGER If a ring is stuck on a swollen finger, save the digit (and the ring!) with paracord. Wrap a length of the internal strand tightly around the finger from the nail upward, tuck the free end under the ring, and tug slowly. The material's stretchiness compresses tissues; the smooth weave helps pull the band down with less friction.

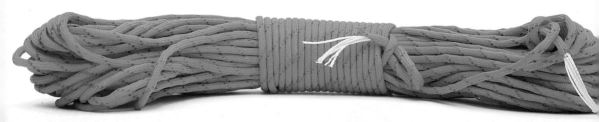

33 TIE THREE USEFUL KNOTS

You can read entire books on knots and practice all of the complicated ones, but you really only need to know a few basic knots to get by. If you can't remember how to tie a knot, no matter how fancy or useful, it's useless. Focus on learning a few basic knots to use for a variety of needs. Here are three basic ones that are easy to master.

SET UP A SQUARE KNOT This is a classic for connecting two lines. Whether you're tying a pair of ropes together to make a single longer one, or bundling firewood to carry, a square knot is a sure winner, and it's also much more secure and stable than its cousin, the granny. You can tie it just by lapping right over left, then left over right.

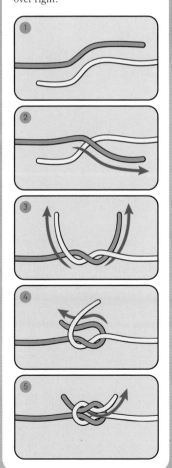

TIE TWO HALF HITCHES This knot is great for attaching line to a tree or pole, hanging hammocks, and securing tarps for shelters. Wrap the free end around the standing end to make the first half hitch, then wrap it around in the same direction again for the second. Pull tight and you have two half hitches; an overhand knot in the free end keeps it from slipping.

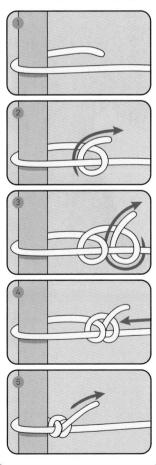

BUILD A BOWLINE The "king of knots" is secure, can be tied one-handed, and won't stick no matter the load it's handed. It can be used as a snare, a rescue line, and more. Tie an overhand loop in your rope, then pull the working end through it from beneath. Circle it behind the rope above the loop, then back through the loop, then pull to tighten.

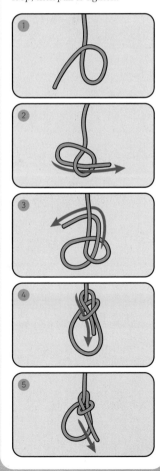

34 DEFEND YOURSELF

In the space between good situational awareness and choosing to carry a weapon is the realm of unarmed self-defense. Even the best of situational awareness can fail, and not everyone wants to carry a less-than-lethal weapon or a gun; for those people, a set of defense techniques represents a better option. And in tactical situations you want to have as many choices as possible; even if you choose to carry something for self-defense, learning a martial art as well is both responsible and smart.

35 GET SCHOOLED

While you can learn a few basic techniques from watching videos online or reading a book, choosing a school to practice with is one of the most important decisions you'll make. There are a lot martial arts types to choose from, and some people will have strong opinions about which of them is "best" for you. It is very true that there are advantages and disadvantages to every martial art, but there is one decision that is more important than that—namely, which martial art looks fun to you? If you're not having fun, you're not likely to keep at it. The style you pick may not be the most aggressive or optimal for street fighting, but it's unlikely you will face people with real martial arts skills, so you will still have a significant advantage. Besides, life is too short to pick up a practice that you don't also enjoy.

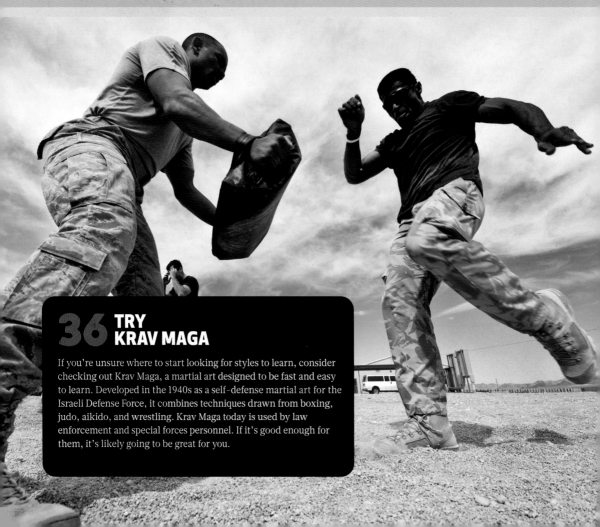

36 TRY KRAV MAGA

If you're unsure where to start looking for styles to learn, consider checking out Krav Maga, a martial art designed to be fast and easy to learn. Developed in the 1940s as a self-defense martial art for the Israeli Defense Force, it combines techniques drawn from boxing, judo, aikido, and wrestling. Krav Maga today is used by law enforcement and special forces personnel. If it's good enough for them, it's likely going to be great for you.

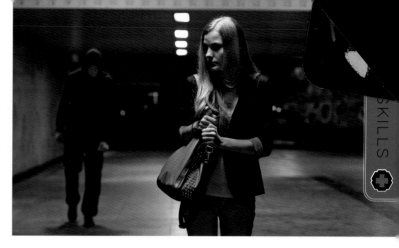

37 KEEP AT IT

For self-defense techniques to be effective, you have to pick a style and practice, practice, practice. Practice is important in order to develop muscle memory, which allows you to react without any hesitation while under attack. Without practice, you quickly lose the ability to perform those skills competently, leaving you in a situation worse than if you had chosen to run away instead.

You should consider martial arts to be a part of your regular workout routine—something you do every week to stay fit and ready. One- or two-day classes offer very limited long-term results because they don't offer the reinforcement that regular training provides. That said, a set of short-term classes do offer you two benefits: the opportunity to decide if you want to explore the style further, and supplemental training to what you're already learning. Some training is better than no training, but regular training is still the best.

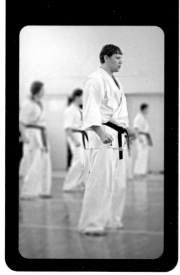

38 USE YOUR IMAGINATION

One of the worst things that can happen if you are being attacked is that you freeze up and do nothing. Usually this happens because the person has no training and has been confronted by a set of circumstances that he or she hasn't encountered before. Martial arts training may eventually provide you with the ability to defend yourself against attack, but you have another tool you can use to prepare yourself: mental visualization and rehearsal. This technique has been proven to help people react more effectively by providing virtual mental training for circumstances that you can't easily simulate. This won't replace any actual training, but it can still enhance your performance and your reaction times. Visualization works, because when you imagine responding to a situation appropriately and quickly, you are also creating neural patterns in your brain just as if you'd physically performed the action. As with any other training method, visualization needs to be repeated; schedule regular sessions to practice the circumstances you feel you most want to home in on.

RELAX AND FOCUS Take a couple of deep breaths and close your eyes, preferably in a quiet place where nobody will bother you.

SET THE SCENE Say that you want to practice responding to a pickpocket or someone trying to snatch your purse. Visualize the environment where it'll take place. Are you alone on the street or in a crowded market? Imagine the scenario taking place in different environments so as not to create a rigid model in your mind.

IMAGINE THE MOMENT Once the stage is set, imagine someone approaching you and making a grab. You'll likely be surprised in real life; imagine being briefly surprised by the attempt but quickly taking control of your actions and awareness.

REACT TO IT Quickly scan for threats or weapons, then grab your stuff back. Yell, "Help, mugger!" as loud as you can and, if the assailant doesn't release your things, push, elbow, and knee them until he lets go. Visualize being confident, strong, and winning the fight.

HANDLE THE AFTERMATH Imagine getting to a safe place immediately afterward and then contacting the police to report the crime.

END THE SCENARIO Now, release the mental image, letting it slowly fade. When you're ready, open your eyes.

39
DO WHAT IT TAKES

If, despite all your best efforts, you end up in a situation with no self-defense training, and yet you must defend yourself, then you're now in a hard situation where you must adapt and overcome.

Studies show that those who have a strong will and don't give up can do much better in a situation such as this. If you're going in to fight, then fight hard, and do it to win. But also fight for the right reasons. If somebody is stealing your phone, it's probably not worth it to start a confrontation, but if your life or the life of a loved one is at risk, then do whatever it takes for you to be victorious.

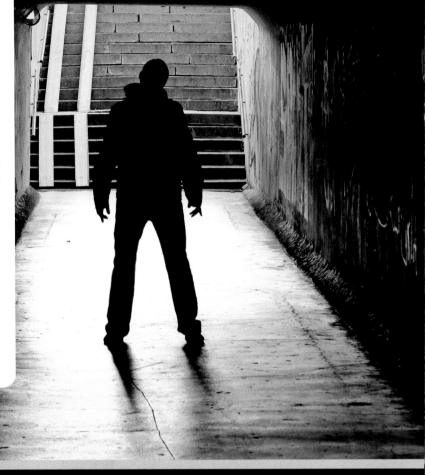

40 AVOID KNIFE FIGHTS

Most people who carry a knife think that it ups their chances for survival in, well, a knife fight. But movies about 1950s gangs aside, odds are slim that you'll end up in an alley with knife-wielding thugs looking to rumble. If you do find yourself in a knife fight, you'll probably only realize it after you've been stabbed.

In most cases, you won't have time to draw your knife, and someone armed with one is unlikely to give you time to level the playing field. If they already have the drop on you, think defensively because, unless you're skilled at knife fighting, it's gonna get messy.

If fact, don't think of it as a "fight" at all. Fights with weapons escalate and end quickly. If a knife is your best option, then act fast before your adversary has a chance, because he or she will likely attack unpredictably. Even if you "win," you'll likely emerge with serious injuries yourself and, depending on the circumstances, such wounds could be fatal. Since most knife-fighting techniques evolved from martial arts, unless you're proficient in that art your best defense is running away instead of drawing a weapon.

41 HIT WHERE IT COUNTS

Where to aim those punches? Target the most fragile areas of your attacker's body with a fist or elbow strike; you might stun him long enough to get away. Follow through on each strike, as if aiming for a point just beyond your attacker. This ensures that you transfer the most power into each and every blow. Follow up with more strikes until he or she is overwhelmed, runs away, or gives in. Here are some sweet spots.

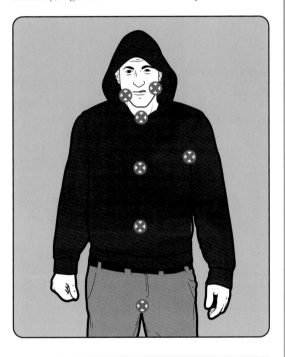

- Below ear
- Side of neck
- Base of throat
- Solar plexus
- Armpit
- Lower abs
- Groin

42 THROW A POWER PUNCH

If you have to punch someone, make it count. The difference between a power punch and a weak swat can mean ending a fight quickly or getting beaten up. If you want to pack a wallop, follow these steps.

STEP 1 Choose a target. You can hit any part of the body, but you won't always have time to select the ideal spot. The good news is that your adversary comes prepackaged with a perfectly centered target: the base of the throat. A well-landed blow will make him gasp for air and momentarily stun him.

STEP 2 Remember your feet; throwing a punch will depend on a solid stance. If you're right-handed, stand with your feet shoulder width apart, your left foot forward, and your body turned at an angle to the attacker. For lefties, reverse it. Your back leg should support your weight.

STEP 3 Put your weight behind the punch instead of just using your arm strength. Push off of your back foot and, as your arm uncoils, swivel your torso to drive your arm. As your punch extends, shift your weight forward to your front foot, which should come naturally.

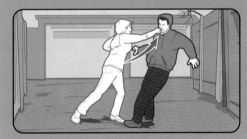

43 SHOUT IT OUT

Whatever's going wrong, if you really need assistance then call for it properly. It's reflexive to just yelp "Hey!" if someone snatches your purse or your phone and makes a run for it, but to get attention, call for it right. If you've been mugged, yell "THIEF!" If there's something burning, take a deep breath and shout "FIRE!" Calling specific attention to the problem at hand will hopefully get more attention drawn to it.

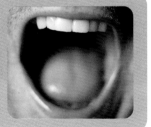

44 STOCK YOUR TOOLSHED

No matter what advertisers may want you to believe, there's no one tool that will get you out of every jam. But if you stock up on these essentials, you'll be well set to face a multitude of issues.

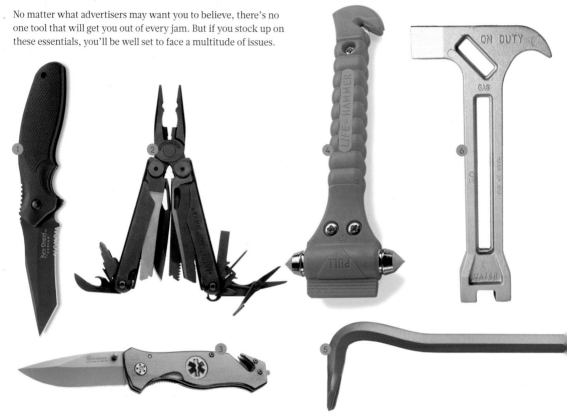

TACTICAL KNIFE While hopefully you won't have to protect yourself from attackers, it could happen, and there's no harm in having a good self-defense knife just in case. This sort of knife is sometimes used as a backup to firearms by those in the military and law enforcement. They're rugged and relatively large, with a razor-sharp blade.

MULTITOOL The versatile multitool got its start as the venerable Swiss Army knife and has a wide number of fold-out tools including screwdrivers, pliers, saws, and knife blades. Though it's not as effective as a fully stocked toolbox, it's a great deal easier to carry with you.

RESCUE KNIFE Also known as an EMS knife, this handy tool is commonly carried by all manner of emergency services personnel, from firefighters to police to paramedics. It's a folding knife with a blade that's at least partly serrated and features two very important accessories: a seat-belt cutter and a window breaker. If you don't wear it on your belt, keep one in your car.

RESCUE TOOL If you prefer not to keep a knife in your car, then this rescue tool can help you escape from your own vehicle after an accident as well as allowing you to help free others who may be in peril. It's designed to be

mounted inside your vehicle for easy access, and it will break side and rear windows easily and cut seat belts safely.

CROW BAR This is the epitome of a tool that you may not use all that often but you will be glad to have one when you need it. In disasters they are primarily used for forcing locks, doors and windows open after being damaged, as well as for various secondary uses such as clearing debris, prying apart boards, removing nails, and even self-defense.

UTILITY SHUT-OFF TOOL While you can use regular household tools to shut off your utilities in a pinch,

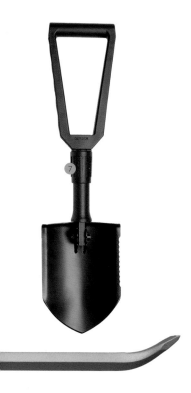

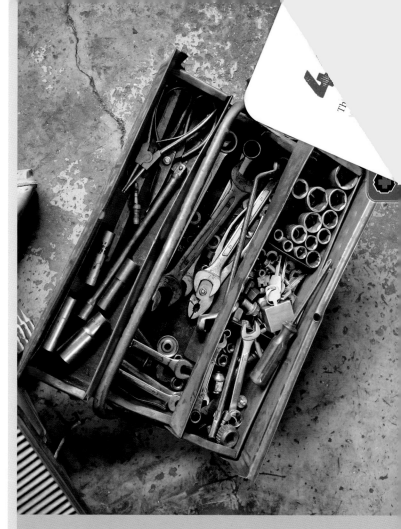

having a combined tool makes it really easy to grab and go or include in your disaster tool kit. Not only does this non-sparking tool allow you to shut off your gas and water, it can also be used to do some light rescue work, such as prying open doors and breaking windows.

7 **FOLDING SHOVEL** Also called an entrenching tool, these compact spades were originally designed for military use. However, there are a myriad of civilian uses for disasters, winter, camping, and self-defense. Those that have a serrated edge can also be used as a saw. The ability to dig latrines is of special note in disasters when water is scarce or unavailable.

45 FILL YOUR HOUSEHOLD TOOL KIT

Even if you're not the handy type who likes to fix things, you should still consider having a basic hand tool kit in your home. It's better to have a tool and never use it than need a tool and not have it. During a disaster or in an emergency you may not have the ability to go buy tools, so having a kit handy becomes an extension of your emergency kit. And who knows, you might also be able to fix something with the tools now that you have them. Household tool kits are often sold in complete packages with a storage case. A good general tool kit includes the following.

- Hammer/mallet
- Saw
- Screwdrivers (Phillips and flat, in various sizes)
- Razor knife
- Wrenches (adjustable and open end, in various sizes)
- Hex keys (in various sizes)
- Wire cutter/stripper
- Pliers (slip-joint and groove-joint)
- Needle-nose pliers
- Digital voltmeter
- Tape measure
- Level

6 CHOOSE A BASIC SELF-PROTECTION GUN

re are many different considerations for whether you
ant to own a gun and, if so, what kind. If you're planning
to purchase your first firearm, and you're not sure what to
buy, consider buying a revolver. While they're slower to load
and lack the convenience of semiautomatic magazines, but
they have some unique benefits.

First off, revolvers are easier to for beginners to learn and
reliably operate than a semi-automatic handgun. Also, they
can be easily fired one handed. Avoid guns that require both
hands, in case you've injured one arm and you can't safely
or accurately use one.

Several common revolvers can be loaded with different
calibers of ammunition. A .357 Magnum, for example, can
be loaded with a lighter .38 Special round if the
shooter is less experienced, or unwilling to deal
with the stronger recoil of a magnum round. In
addition, any revolver can fire a wide range of
different loads, from snake shot to self-
defense, without the feed problems a
semiautomatic has. If you want more
capcity, seven- or eight-shot revolvers
are available give you more capacity than
the old fashioned "six-shooter."

These guns can be easier to conceal,
especially when open-carrying a weapon
in an urban environment can make you
an instant target. Most importantly,
revolvers are less likely to malfunction,
especially in the hands of a
less experienced user in a
high stress situation.

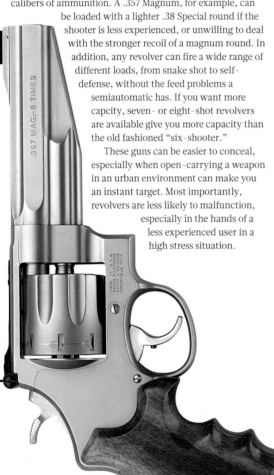

47 HANDLE GUNS SAFELY

Regardless if you have a lot of training or have
never picked up a gun before in your life,
reviewing and knowing these basic gun-safety
rules can make the difference between safely
handling a gun and an accidental discharge.

ASSUME EVERY GUN IS LOADED Every time you
see a gun, pick up a gun, or point a gun, you
should assume that it's loaded. Even if someone
unloaded it right in front of you, continue to
treat it as if it's loaded.

ONLY POINT YOUR GUN AT A TARGET Even if the
gun is unloaded, never point the muzzle at
anything you are not willing to destroy.

KEEP YOUR HANDS TO YOURSELF Do not touch
the trigger until the sights are on-target.

BE SURE OF YOUR TARGET Be absolutely sure
that you are shooting at what you're intending to
hit and that there are no bystanders anywhere
near it. Never shoot at a sound or movement.

HAVE A SAFE BACKSTOP Look beyond your
target before you make your shot. High-
powered ammunition can travel up to a mile.

CARRY SAFELY Make sure the safety is on and
that the barrel is pointing down when you are
walking with your gun.

CLIMB CAREFULLY Do not climb up a tree or over
a fence with a loaded gun. Hand your gun to a
partner with the safety on and have them hand
it back to you when you're done.

SHOOT SOBER Never mix drinking and guns.

CHECK IT OUT Before you use any new or
borrowed equipment, go over everything and
make sure that it is working properly. Be sure
you know how everything operates before you
attempt to use it.

STORE SAFELY Store and transport ammo
separate from guns, and keep everything under
lock and key when not in use.

48 CARRY RESPONSIBLY

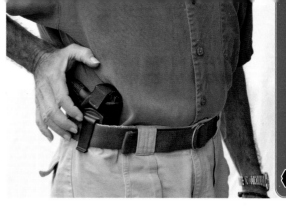

The best personal-protection gun is the one you never have to use. A permit to carry a concealed handgun is just that—a permit to carry it. It's not a permit to use it. Handgun use is covered by laws dealing with self-defense, and those laws apply whether you are carrying a handgun or not.

A gun carries the power of life and death. The responsible concealed carrier will act with greater calm and wisdom than an unarmed person. That means you have to hold yourself to a higher standard, with brandishing your weapon being your last line of defense, not your first. Good situational awareness and knowing how to avoid confrontations before they become potentially violent remain the best approach.

Weapons have the power to end violent confrontations. You may come out alive but the cost of doing so may be high,

as you may temporarily lose your liberty, be sued in civil court, incur expensive legal bills, and be put on trial in the court of public opinion. Risk these things when it matters, such as defending yourself from imminent and significant danger; anything less than that simply isn't worth it.

49 ZAP A BAD GUY

In the self-defense arsenal, between guns and pepper spray, we find tasers and stun guns. While some people use these terms interchangeably for less-than-lethal electrical weapons, they are different types of device.

Ⓐ TASERS This tool shoots barbed electrodes at an assailant, allowing you to use them at a distance—15 feet (4.5 meters) in the case of civilian models.

Ⓑ STUN GUNS By contrast, to use a stun gun you have to be very close to your assailant, as the device is handheld and requires direct physical contact.

Either can be a good option, but ideally you'll have other methods of defense as well, used in a continuum of force options rather than as a sole source of defense. That said, as a last-ditch tool they can be useful to briefly incapacitate your opponent so that you can safely escape.

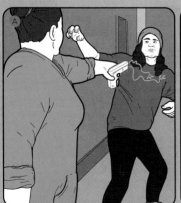
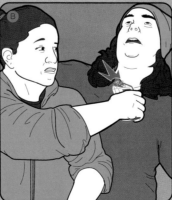

50 WIELD PEPPER SPRAY

If you feel the need for a self-defense tool that's not as serious a commitment as a gun or knife, consider getting pepper spray. Depending on the canister type you buy, they can offer about a 10- to 15-foot (3-4.5 meters) range, and they carry enough juice to discharge multiple bursts. Hollywood has also skewed the perception of how effective pepper spray is—it may not always deter an assailant, and you risk contaminating yourself as much as you might slow down an assailant. Consider taking a class taught by a self-defense school or the local police department to be sure that you use this tool as effectively as possible.

51 LIGHT IT UP

Darkness is inevitable. Seeing in the dark is a choice. The solution: a flashlight—or flashlights—because you will likely want one wherever you are. I own several flashlights: one for each car, one for everyday carry, one by my bed, one for work, and quite a few more, but you get the idea. Fenix is a longtime leader in the business of high-quality, yet affordable, tactical flashlights. For everyday emergency user I recommend the Fenix PD35 TAC Tactical Edition, which balances size, power, run time, quality, and price. When choosing a tactical flashlight, consider these traits, and make your best choice accordingly:

A tactical flashlight needs to be small enough to be easily and unobtrusively carried—generally, no larger than the size of your extended palm.

Your flashlight needs to operate in all weather and handle immersion in water, so consider one that is rated IP67 or IP68; a good flashlight will last decades and endure harsh conditions. Hard anodized aluminum is tough yet light, making for a solid, reliable body.

Choose a model with a LED bulb. Incandescent bulbs break easily, burn out unexpectedly, and are no where near as bright; modern LEDs are comparably indestructible and are more efficient, giving you brighter light and longer runtimes.

To be effective as a self-defense tool (by temporarily blinding and disorienting an attacker in the dark) a flashlight needs to be extremely bright and feature a strobe mode. Modern LEDs emit 1,000 or more lumens (the measurement of the total visible light emitted by a source), but anything over 600 is acceptable.

Consider a flashlight with both a high-output setting for self-defense and a low-output mode for longer battery life in everyday use.

Opt for a model that can use either regular batteries or rechargeable. Regular batteries can be used to quickly swap out your primary rechargeable battery without having to wait for the rechargeable battery to recharge.

Lastly, for use as a last-ditch self-defense weapon—consider one with a toothed or strike bezel.

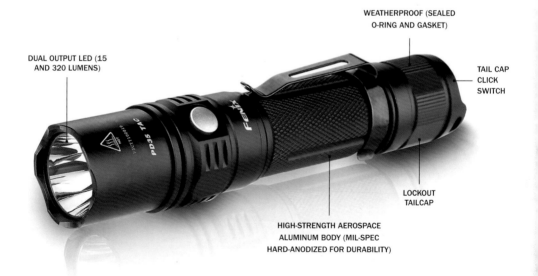

WEATHERPROOF (SEALED O-RING AND GASKET)

DUAL OUTPUT LED (15 AND 320 LUMENS)

TAIL CAP CLICK SWITCH

LOCKOUT TAILCAP

HIGH-STRENGTH AEROSPACE ALUMINUM BODY (MIL-SPEC HARD-ANODIZED FOR DURABILITY)

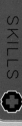

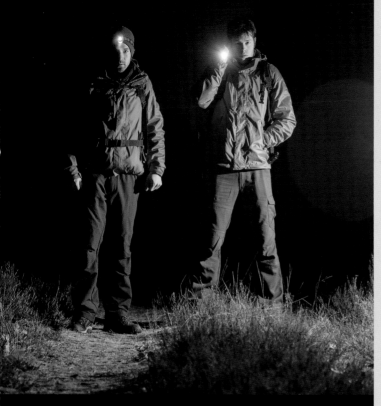

53 GET A HEADLIGHT

Along with regular flashlights, another tool that you should include in your go bag is an LED headlamp. These are very useful for several reasons: They keep your hands free, they're designed for long battery life on regular AAA batteries, and they offer a wide variety of settings; some models even have a low-power red LED that preserves night vision and provides even longer battery life. When you realize how useful headlamps are for all manner of household tasks, or changing tires at the side of the road, or while camping, you'll wonder how you survived so long without several of them.

52 SHINE BRIGHT

There are lots of tactical uses for a flashlight. Here are the most common situations in which you may find a good flashlight to be indispensable.

BE A FIREFLY To move with more stealth, briefly switch your light on to scan the area and your path before proceeding a short distance in the dark. Repeat as necessary until you get to safety.

IDENTIFY FRIEND OR FOE Use your light to verify that an area is clear and, if you spot someone, to see if he or she is armed or not.

DETER ANIMALS Most animals will freeze and then usually run away when blinded by bright light.

BLIND YOUR OPPONENT Shine the light into an attacker's eyes, then give yourself enough time to flee or to get the upper hand if you need to fight.

LIGHT YOUR SIGHTS If you're carrying a firearm, you can use the "eye index" technique by holding the light up to the side of your head in order to illuminate both your target and your weapon sights.

DEFEND YOURSELF Flashlights aren't considered weapons, so they can be carried almost anywhere and used as a last-ditch bludgeon if all else fails.

54 WARD OFF WATER

The current set of ANSI FL1 standards for flashlights has three water-resistance levels. Knowing the strength of each rating will help you decide the best light for you.

IPX4
Splashing water such as rain

IPX7
Submerged to 1 meter for 30 minutes

IPX8
Submerged deeper than 1 meter for up to 4 hours

55 RUN ON SUNLIGHT

During an emergency or disaster it's common to lose power for extended periods of time—sometimes even weeks. Considering how often we rely on portable devices, a small solar generator allows you to keep using your critical devices long past spare battery packs have died.

I recommend the Goal Zero Yeti series of portable generators. Not only can they charge using a variety of fixed and portable solar panels, they will also charge from AC wall power, along with 12-volt power from most vehicles and vessels.

This generator system has an easy-to-use, informative display and replaceable batteries. It is also chainable to other batteries, so the main unit can extend its capacity. It has five to 10 different output ports (depending on model), to provide a variety of power options for 12 volt, USB, and AC. You won't need fuel to operate it (thus making it safe to use indoors), and it's silent since it does not use a noisy internal combustion system to generate power.

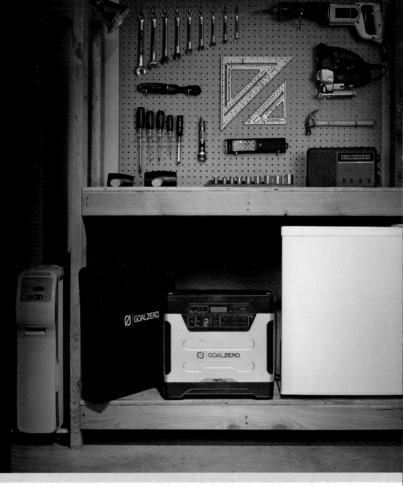

56 GET POWER IN YOUR POCKET

When you're on the move, you might not be able to bring a larger power supply or charging system with you. Under those circumstances, you will need a portable solution that can be stored in your go bag.

Depending on your individual situation and needs, this handy device might even be considered useful as an everyday carry item—for instance, if you're spending a lot of time in the field away from opportunities to charge your electronics.

Additionally, a portable charger can be useful for when you go camping, hiking, or do other outdoor recreational activities.

Solar chargers that have carabiners or mounting straps are easily attached to your backpack or go bag so that it can work in daylight while you go about your business. You also want to have multiple USB ports, the ability to also charge from AC power, good-quality battery cells and solar panels, and a fuel gauge to show how much power is left in reserve. Some models also have built-in fault indicators, and flashlights run by the unit's internal power.

Pocket models aren't much bigger than a tube of lipstick and can carry enough power for a full charge on a mobile phone (depending on your model). Just remember to keep it fully charged so that, when you need it, there will be power aplenty to charge your devices.

57 HACK A VEHICLE BATTERY FOR POWER

While not a long-term solution for the loss of the power grid, this DIY battery system can charge critical electronic devices to give you more than a week's worth of use. Sometimes, just having access to a limited yet reliable power supply can make a big difference.

If you want to use this system indoors, use an absorbed glass mat (AGM) battery; the traditional lead-acid types can produce harmful fumes. You can purchase a 55 AH (ampere-hour) 12-volt battery from home-improvement or boating stores, or repurpose one from a boat, RV, or other vehicle. You can order batteries with even more capacity, but size and cost will both increase. You will also need a battery wall charger, a cigarette lighter adapter, a cell phone car charger, and a voltmeter to test the setup.

Wear safety goggles and take great care when working with batteries. AGM batteries are less toxic than lead-acid car batteries but still contain acid.

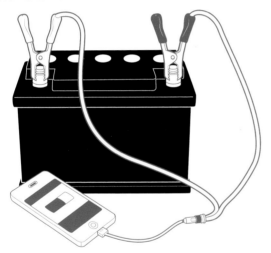

STEP 1 Using the voltmeter, ensure that your battery is fully charged. If you store your battery, check up on it every three months. If the charge drops below 12.4 volts, charge it so it'll be ready to go when the lights go out. A smart charger with an automatic trickle charge mode will keep the battery fully charged for when you need it.

STEP 2 Attach the cigarette lighter port to your battery. It's easy—the port attaches to wires with a set of jumper cable-like alligator clips.

STEP 3 Plug in the phone charger, as you would in your car, and charge up your phone. Your results will vary based on the number and capacity of the devices that you're charging, and the total capacity of the battery, but modern smartphones will recharge about 25 times with your typical fully charged car battery—more so for those larger-capacity marine batteries.

STEP 4 Periodically insert the voltmeter into the cigarette lighter adapter to check on your voltage—you don't want to run your battery down too far. As when it's in storage, never let it drop below 12.4 volts.

58 UNDERSTAND BATTERY CAPACITY

The milliampere-hour, abbreviated to mAH, is a unit of electrical charge frequently used to rate the capacity of batteries. In order to understand how large a battery you need to charge one or more of your devices, add up each device's battery mAH and compare it to the battery that you are using to charge them. You'll have a good approximation of how many charges you have left in your battery before needing to recharge. Ideally, you'll want a battery that fully charges the intended device to at least 80% or better. For those looking at large batteries, 1 AH = 1000 mAH.

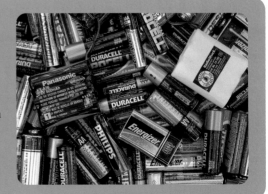

59 IMPROVISE A FIRST AID KIT

It's almost inevitable that you'll run out of some medical supplies no matter how well stocked your kit is. Making use of common household items for first aid is a good way to extend the supplies you do have or to provide aid in circumstances when you don't have a proper kit on hand. Take a moment to look through your kitchen, bathroom, bedroom, and garage and note how you might be able to use what you already have in your house for first aid.

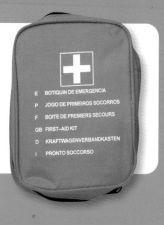

60 GO TO BEDROOM, BATHROOM, AND BEYOND

Chances are, you have a fair amount of first-aid supplies loose in your bathroom and maybe packed away in a travel kit for when you go on the road. Consider consolidating all of those supplies into one place such as a box or a backpack so that you can easily move the supplies or inventory them when needed.

PACK YOUR SOCKS Instead of Coban or Kerlex, tube socks can be cut to create a bandage cover. Just take a clean sock and cut the foot portion off. Now you can use the "sleeve" to hold bandages in place [A], which is especially useful when having to move a lot after being bandaged.

EXPAND YOUR SPANDEX If you cut a lycra shirt torso into a spiral, or simply cut the sleeve or leg from a lycra garment, you'll have various lengths of stretch material that can be used in place of Ace bandages to stabilize sprains or strains, or to tie splints in place [B].

GRAB A BANDANA Use a bandana or any square scarf as an arm sling [C]. Regular scarves can be used to secure the sling to the torso more comfortably than a belt.

TAMP DOWN BLEEDING While they are not ideally used for treating severe trauma such as gunshot wounds, tampons and sanitary napkins can be a stand-in for proper trauma dressings and are clean and absorbent. Additional uses include pads as eyepatches or splint padding, and slim tampons for nosebleeds [D].

GET SALTY Epsom salts can be used for many different purposes beyond first aid, so keeping a supply at home is just a good idea in general. For first aid, epsom salts can be used to treat or sooth bites, stings, sunburns, poison ivy [E], blisters, and even as a laxative.

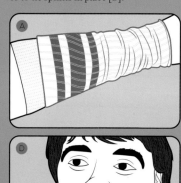

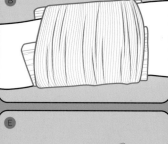

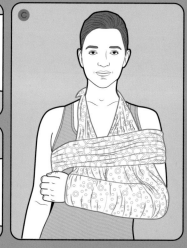

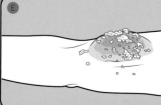

61 RAID YOUR KITCHEN

If you find yourself low on first-aid supplies, you can also consider using a wide variety of kitchen and household goods to substitute. They're not the perfect tools for the job, but they'll do in a pinch.

1 **KEEP YOUR SPIRITS UP** 120 proof or stronger spirits can disinfect equipment or hands, but you should not clean wounds with it unless there's no alternative. Drinking alcohol isn't the best thing for pain management, but it's better than nothing.

2 **COVER BURNS** Plastic wrap can be used for partial- and full-thickness thermal burns (though unnecessary for superficial burns and not to be used for chemical burns). After the skin has cooled, apply a single layer directly to the wound with no ointment, and secure it loosely with gauze.

3 **BAG YOUR HANDS** Preventing the spread of disease and isolation from infectious body fluids is a basic part of medicine. If you run out of medical gloves, use a plastic bag as a crude mitten. It's a little unwieldy but better than nothing.

4 **SOOTHE WITH VINEGAR** Vinegar is a natural antiseptic and, diluted 50-50 with water, can clean minor cuts and abrasions. The same solution can also reduce itching from poison ivy or insect bites, and soothe sunburns with a soaked towel laid on the skin or applied directly with a spray bottle.

5 **EMPLOY SAFETY PINS** Seemingly a common item found in first aid kits, you'd be surprised at how many have none. You can hold bandages in place with these, and they're also good for digging out splinters.

6 **TENDERIZE STINGS** Many unflavored meat tenderizers contain the enzyme papain, which breaks down proteins, thus diminishing the pain and discomfort associated with venom from stings. Don't leave tenderizer on skin for more than 10 to 15 minutes, as it can cause an irritating reaction itself.

7 **HEAL WITH BAKING SODA** You can stop stinging, itching, and swelling from insect bites by applying a paste of soda and water on the affected area. To relieve heartburn, indigestion, or upset stomach, dissolve a half-teaspoon of baking soda in a half-glass of water, and drink every few hours as needed.

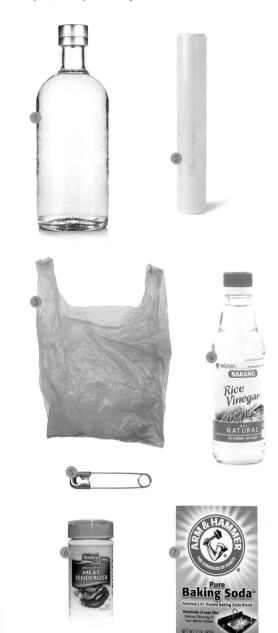

62 FILL UP YOUR FIRST AID KIT

Ideally, you'll have a fully stocked first aid kit handy when a medical emergency strikes. However, if you need to improvise, a range of household objects can do double duty in a pinch.

EYE PATCH Not only for pirates, it protects your eye after an injury and blocks light that can exacerbate migraines.

CHEST TRAUMA SEAL Used to treat severe penetrating injuries to the chest that have punctured the lungs.

TOURNIQUET A last-ditch measure, but tourniquets can be crucial in stopping life-threatening bleeding.

SLING This simple rig allows your arm and shoulder to rest and recover from a range of injuries or strains.

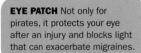

RING CUTTER This handy device can safely remove a ring from a swollen or broken finger. It's a standard ER item.

BANDAGE A bandage is one of your more basic first-aid items; it protects injuries from infection and controls bleeding.

BANDAGE STRIPS For longer wounds, bandage strips work like stitches, sealing the wound closed.

SPLINT Just what the doctor ordered, to stabilizes strains, sprains, and fractures.

IMPROVISED

EYE PATCH If you need to protect an injured eye and don't have an eye patch, try using a folded-up a sanitary pad.

CHEST TRAUMA SEAL Use tape and plastic wrap (sealed only on three sides) to protect an open chest wound.

SLING Scarves make excellent slings—your main goal is just to be sure that the arm is stable and held close to the body.

TOURNIQUET A stick and a length of rope can be used to improvise a tourniquet. Only do this in life-or-death situations.

FINGER WRAP Wrap a piece of dental floss (or paracord—see item 32) under the rings and ease it off the injured finger

BANDAGE Superglue, if applied correctly, can help to safely seal a cut (see item 92).

BANDAGE STRIPS Tape can be used to hold a bandage in place or seal a wound (see item 28).

SPLINT Anything rigid like a cane or a hockey stick can be used to stabilize an injury. Tie it on firmly, or use duct tape.

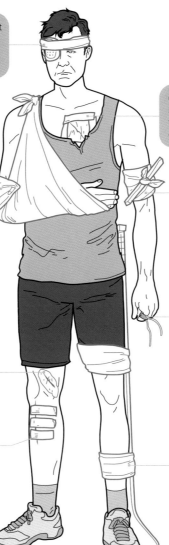

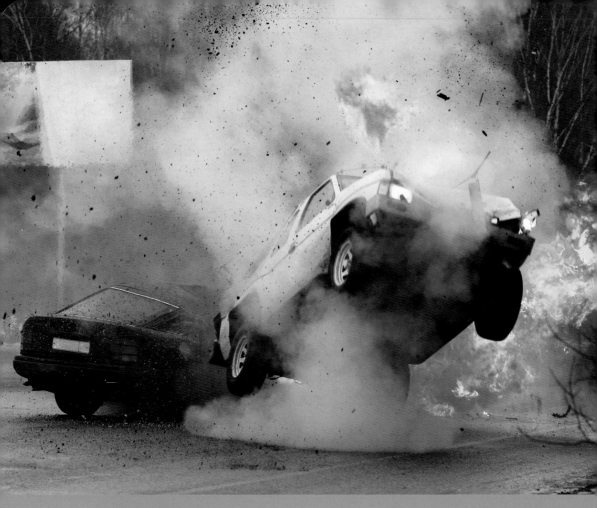

63 BE SAFE ON THE SCENE

In addition to situational awareness, there are some special considerations for your own safety and that of others when offering help in an emergency. "Tunnel vision" can cause regular folks and even first responders to risk their own safety unintentionally. If you determine the scene is unsafe, you may not actually be able to help. Choosing to step back and maintain your own safety when someone is hurt or in danger is never an easy decision, but if you endanger yourself, the risk is that you end up another victim. When you're approaching an incident, look out for various hazards, no matter where it has taken place.

ESTABLISH AREA SAFETY Avoid unstable or dangerous conditions whenever possible and be cautious of any fast-moving vehicle traffic or machinery close to the patient, or any fire, smoke, or chemical exposures in the area.

CHECK FOR WEAPONS Look for anything within reach, in plain view, or held by others possibly hostile people.

LOOK UP Check for hazards from above, especially after earthquakes. There could be risk of falling rocks, furniture at risk for tipping over, or an unstable building.

BEWARE ANIMALS Are there any scared or injured animals near the area?

AVOID ELECTRICITY Damaged electronics, power cords, and power lines should all be considered charged and dangerous.

PROTECT YOURSELF Make sure you are wearing the right PPE for the conditions (see item 25).

64 GET EDUCATED

You can learn basic first aid from books and smartphone apps, but proper training is still best. Courses are available from various organizations; check the Red Cross, your local fire department, junior colleges, and community centers. Your next question is: "What classes should I take?" That will depend on your free time, personal interest, and needs.

Ideally you should have advanced first aid, CPR, and AED (automated external defibrillator) training. If you're short on time, a regular first aid class and an abbreviated hands-only CPR class is a good alternative. If you have pets, a pet first aid class may help you get your four-legged friends through times when you can't get to a vet clinic.

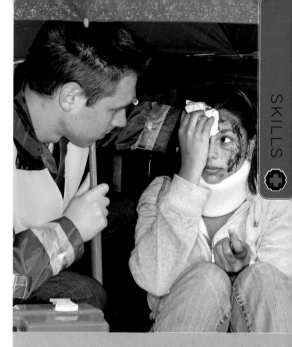

65 GET SOME SERIOUS TRAINING

If you want to dive deep into medical training, here are a few choices, each of which will give you a different set of tools.

BE A FIRST RESPONDER Emergency medical response (EMR) training is the shortest and easiest to complete. It's useful for those who want to focus on immediate emergencies, in support of emergency medical services (EMS) in disasters or smaller events.

GET TECHNICAL Emergency medical technician (EMT) courses are more comprehensive, focusing on geriatric issues, ambulance operations, and equipment you're unlikely to have in your home. This course is more applicable to those interested in volunteering with EMS or having a broad set of skills past immediate first aid.

GO WILD Wilderness EMT training is a great option for those who go camping, hiking, or otherwise spend lots of time in remote wilderness. The skills learned in this class emphasize improvising and helping others with a minimum of resources. However, this class is the most time consuming.

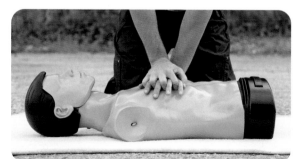

66 TREAT YOUR PATIENTS RIGHT

Regardless of training, one of the most important skills to use, whether treating someone who has a minor scrape or a life-threatening injury, is to help make them feel comforted and safe. But this isn't a technique you'll learn in a first-aid class. It's about approaching an injured person as one human who cares about another. Injured patients are often scared and confused, sometimes in ways that are not immediately obvious.

Reassuring your patient is simple: Tell them that they are safe, that you are there to help them, and that responders are on the way. It may also help to explain what's happening around and to them. You might have to overstate the obvious, but if a patient is in shock, they might be overwhelmed by events. Your calm narration will reduce their anxiety, and their experience of the trauma can be more easily handled. It's one of those moments when you really get to be the hero that makes the difference.

Focus on using positive statements that are true and applicable to the circumstances. For example, somebody who is trapped under a beam after an earthquake is hard to reassure when you don't know how soon responders will get there or when the next aftershock will happen. Circumstances can be challenging, and doing your best will go a long way to helping the injured person know that they are in good hands.

67 BUILD YOUR FIRST AID KIT

Most people think a first aid kit has a few Band-Aids, some aspirin, and a set of tweezers. But a good first-aid kit should be closer to what a professional might carry. These items will all fit into a small box, and won't cost an arm and a leg—but might save them!

Ⓐ Nonadhesive dressings
Ⓑ Antibacterial ointment
Ⓒ SAM splint
Ⓓ 1-inch (2.5-cm) medical tape
Ⓔ Adhesive bandages, including butterfly strips
Ⓕ Anti-inflammatory drugs
Ⓖ Tweezers
Ⓗ Medical shears (a.k.a. EMT scissors)
Ⓘ Disinfectant towelettes
Ⓙ Aloe vera gel
Ⓚ Arm sling
Ⓛ Gauze roller bandages
Ⓜ Sterile compress
Ⓝ Elastic roller bandages
Ⓞ CPR pocket mask
Ⓟ Medical gloves
Ⓠ Electronic thermometer
Ⓡ Space blanket
Ⓢ Coban
Ⓣ Eye wash
Ⓤ Throat lozenges
Ⓥ Wilderness/travel medical guidebook

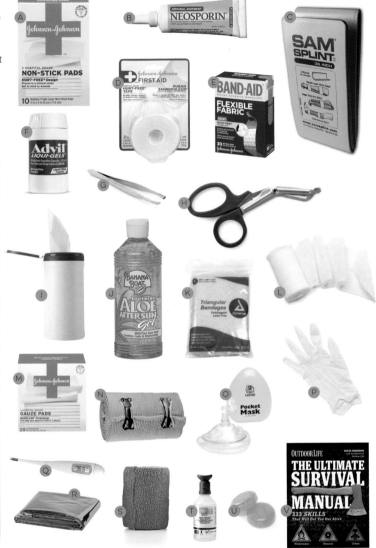

68 TAKE IT TO THE NEXT LEVEL

If you've taken the classes described in item 65, or just have a desire to be even more helpful in a crisis, you might want to add the following items to your stash of medical supplies. If you look for what's called a "jump bag," you'll find that they often come prepacked with these items—and much more!

- BloodStopper bandages
- Chemical cold packs
- Normal saline (for rinsing injuries)
- Oral glucose tablets (for diabetic emergencies)
- Tourniquet
- Stethoscope
- QuikClot (for controlling bleeding)
- Oropharyngeal (OPA) airway kit
- Activated charcoal (for ingested poisons)
- Penlight
- Blood pressure cuff

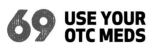

69 USE YOUR OTC MEDS

If you have a prescription that you need in order to survive, that's your number-one concern. But it's also wise to keep a stock of the following over-the-counter medications in your disaster kit.

NAME	PRIMARY USES	OTHER USES	WARNINGS
IBUPROFEN (Motrin, Advil)	Relieves headaches, cramps, earache, sore throat, sinus/muscle/back pain, stiffness/arthritis, and reduces fever; safe for children	—	Increases risk of serious gastrointestinal (GI) bleeding, ulcers, and perforation
ACETAMINOPHEN (Tylenol)	Similar to ibuprofen; generally less effective	—	High doses can cause liver damage
ACETYLSALICYLIC ACID (Aspirin)	Similar to ibuprofen and acetaminophen but used less often	Also treats or prevents heart attack, stroke, and chest pain	Consult medical professionals before use for cardiovascular conditions
LOPERAMIDE (Imodium)	Treats diarrhea, which can be deadly in events where water and medical care are inaccessible	—	—
PSEUDOEPHEDRINE (Sudafed)	Anticongestant, used to treat respiratory infection, allergies, chemical irritation, mild asthma, and bronchitis	Can be used as a stimulant	—
DIPHENHYDRAMINE (Benadryl)	Treats symptoms of allergies or respiratory infections, rashes/hives (such as poison ivy), and nausea	Can also be used as a sleep aid	—
MECLIZINE (Dramamine)	Relieves nausea, vomiting, motion sickness, vertigo, and anxiety	Can also be used as a sleep aid	—
RANITIDINE (Zantac)	Treats heartburn, ulcers, and other stomach issues	Can also relieve hives	—
HYDROCORTISONE (Cortizone 10)	The strongest steroid cream available without a prescription; treats painful or itchy rashes, eczema, poison ivy, diaper rash, and minor skin irritations	—	—
CLOTRIMAZOLE (Gyne-Lotrimin)	Antifungal used to treat athlete's foot, ringworm, and diaper rashes	—	—

70 USE ANTIBIOTICS WISELY

There are a lot of drugs in this category, and while some are broad spectrum, many are only used for specific infections. It's not recommended to use antibiotics without professional medical advice, especially if you have a history of allergic reactions, but having some in your kit can be handy in a disaster. Remember, antibiotics are not antiviral drugs and can't treat flu, colds, coughs, and similar common maladies. You should also finish the entire prescribed amount—stopping when symptoms lessen may create resistant bacteria, and your symptoms can get worse.

NAME	PRIMARY USES	OTHER USES
AMOXICILLIN *(Amoxil)*	Pneumonia, strep throat, ear infections, and salmonella	Sometimes used to treat Lyme disease
LEVOFLOXACIN *(Levaquin)*	Respiratory tract infections, cellulitis, urinary tract infections, anthrax, endocarditis, meningitis, traveler's diarrhea, tuberculosis, plague, and infections that arise after traumatic injuries	——
DOXYCYCLINE *(Periostat)*	Urinary tract infections, chancroid, cholera, Lyme disease, chlamydia, sinusitis, Rocky Mountain spotted fever, bubonic plague, and skin infections	Used to treat MRSA (methycillin-resistant staphylococcus aureus), malaria, and anthrax
AZITHROMYCIN *(Zithromax)*	Pharyngitis, respiratory infections, gastrointestinal infections (such as those caused by eating contaminated food), and chlamydia	——
CEPHALEXIN *(Keflex)*	Ear, bone and joint, skin, and urinary tract infections	May also be used for certain types pneumonia and strep throat
METRONIDAZOLE *(Flagyl)*	Bacterial vaginosis, pelvic inflammatory disease, pseudomembranous colitis, aspiration pneumonia, intra-abdominal infections, lung abscess, gingivitis, amoebiasis, giardiasis, and trichomoniasis	——
CIPROFLOXACIN *(Cipro)*	Wide variety of infections, including infections of bones and joints, gastroenteritis, respiratory tract infections, cellulitis, urinary tract infections, prostatitis, anthrax, and chancroid	——
GENTAMICIN *(Gentasol eyedrops)*	Eye infections	——

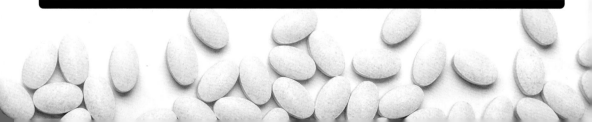

71 KNOW COMMON PRESCRIPTION MEDS

If you can't get medical help in a disaster, knowing what medications do can make a difference. Ideally you should use these only with professional medical advice, as they can be dangerous at the incorrect doses, and some may be addictive or could trigger harmful interactions with other drugs.

FEEL LESS PAIN Plenty of prescription painkillers (many of which combine codeine and acetaminophen) can treat moderate to severe pain. These can help you endure pain that the over-the-counter medications don't handle as well.

TREAT NAUSEA Zofran (ondansetron), a popular antiemetic that comes in a tablet that dissolves under your tongue, can prevent nausea and vomiting caused by morning sickness, heat or dehydration, and other issues.

STAY AWAKE After a disaster you may be fatigued but need to function anyway. Medications such as Provigil (modafinil) and Adderall (amphetamine) are used by various military forces and others to keep them alert and focused. Use cautiously; sooner or later, your sleep debt will need to be paid off with proper rest.

KEEP CALM Stress and anxiety after disaster is common. Benzodiazepines can be an emotional "reset," helping you to avoid panic and function better. Common forms include Valium (diazepam) and Ativan (lorazepam), used to treat anxiety, panic attacks, insomnia, seizures, and muscle spasms. These drugs are addictive; occasional use is acceptable, but regular use is cautioned against.

BREATHE RIGHT Ventolin (albuterol sulfate) inhalers can help an asthmatic or someone suffering from chronic obstructive pulmonary disease (COPD) who is having trouble breathing. Off-label uses include treating difficult breathing associated with respiratory infection.

STOP SERIOUS ALLERGIES EpiPens (epinephrine) are used to treat anaphylaxis—a serious allergic reaction that causes severe swelling and respiratory obstruction—experienced by some people from insect stings, shellfish or peanut allergies.

GO (ANTI) VIRAL Tamiflu (oseltamivir) is used to treat and prevent influenza. Thought somewhat controversial, it may be used in a pandemic to reduce risk of death, especially for at-risk populations such as the immunocompromised or elderly, or within 48 hours of contracting flu symptoms.

STOP RADIATION Potassium iodide (KI) helps to prevent radioactive iodine from being absorbed by the thyroid gland during a radiation incident. People should only take KI if advised by public health or emergency management officials, as there are health risks associated with its use.

KEEP CONTRACEPTION Plan B (levonorgestrel), also called the "morning-after pill," is an OTC drug and can be used up to 72 hours after unprotected sex, a condom failure, or sexual assault. Keeping this in your medical kit may help someone avoid dealing with unwanted pregnancy in the midst of coping with a disaster.

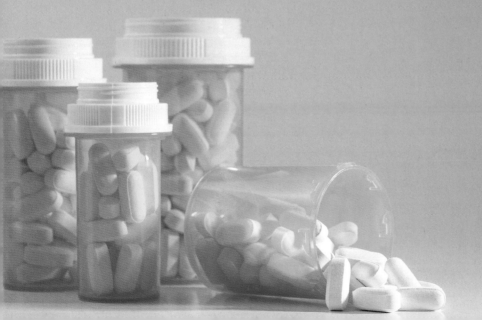

72 KNOW COMMON ALLERGIES

Allergic reactions are generally caused by a few major categories of allergens. Here is an overview of the most common types that may trigger a reaction.

FOOD	DRUG	INSECT/POISON	OTHER
Eggs, fish, milk (not to be confused with lactose intolerance), peanuts, shellfish, soy, tree nuts, wheat	Anticonvulsants, insulin, penicillin, sulfa drugs, and related antibiotics	Fire ants, bees, wasps, hornets, and yellow jackets	Animal dander or hair, mold, dust, latex, cosmetics, and pollens from trees, grasses, or weeds

73 PREPARE FOR ANAPHYLAXIS

Severe allergic reactions from insect stings and other allergens can lead to anaphylaxis, which includes a sudden decrease in blood pressure and difficulty breathing. In extreme instances, the reaction can kill in minutes. Anyone can experience a life-threatening allergic reaction, even if he or she has never had a problem before; other allergies may develop over time and exposure. There are only limited actions you can take in this situation, and you must act early and decisively.

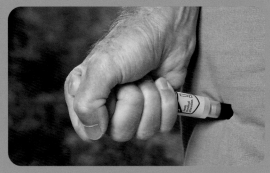

BE PREPARED When traveling or in a disaster, ask all of your companions if they have issues with insect stings or other allergic reactions. If so, find out if they carry an epinephrine auto-injector, such as an EpiPen.

ACT QUICKLY Be alert to the first signs of a serious allergic reaction: skin reactions such as itching (especially around wrists, the insides of elbows, and on the face), hives, pale skin, or swelling of the lips, throat, or anywhere on the face. Beware of constriction of the airway or trouble breathing, wheezing, a weak pulse, or vomiting or nausea. Act at the very first sign of any of these indicators. Do not wait to see if symptoms worsen.

GET HELP Head to emergency medical facilities. If in a remote area or during a disaster, create an evacuation plan: Contact emergency personnel about the potential need for

rescue, and plan on where it will take place. If contact isn't possible, create a plan to transport the person to definitive medical care as quickly as possible.

GIVE FIRST AID Give over-the-counter diphenhydramine such as Benadryl; the liquid form is fastest. This won't stave off a severe case of anaphylaxis alone—it's just a first step. Prepare to perform CPR and rescue breathing if symptoms worsen. Prepare to administer epinephrine via auto-injector if available.

USE EPINEPHRINE If the victim begins to experience trouble breathing, use the epinephrine auto-injector as shown in item 74, and do whatever you can to help get them to medical personnel. Time is absolutely critical here. If necessary, perform CPR and rescue breathing. Administer additional epinephrine if available.

74 EMPLOY AN EPIPEN

While anaphylaxis is uncommon, it can be deadly. Milder reactions can be unpleasant and sometimes a little harmful to the victim, but anaphylactic shock can be lethal if left untreated. This allergic reaction can take place in just a few minutes, with the victim experiencing severe swelling and rashes, difficulty breathing, and dangerous changes in blood pressure and heart rate.

If you know that someone is experiencing this sort of reaction, you can help treat it with epinephrine (medical adrenaline) administered by a penlike auto-injector. If you keep one in your medical kit, make sure it's kept in a stable-temperature environment and is within its expiration date; replace as needed.

STEP 1 Remove injector from the carrying tube and remove the safety cap from the end of the injector.

STEP 2 Grip the shaft firmly, with your thumb on its back. Aim for the thigh or upper arm. (You can even go through a layer of clothing.)

STEP 3 Jab down firmly against the muscle, keeping the shaft of the pen perpendicular to his or her limb. Hold the injector in place for 10 seconds to allow the needle to deploy and the medicine to be administered.

STEP 4 Remove the needle from the victim's limb, and carefully place the injector back into the carrying tube.

STEP 5 Monitor the victim's condition and seek medical attention, as he or she may need additional care after the medication wears off.

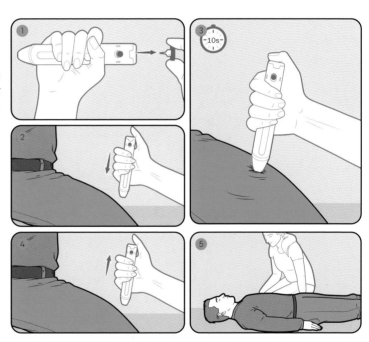

75 LOOK FOR A MEDIC ALERT

If you come across somebody who is unconscious or no longer can speak due to a possible allergic reaction, take a moment to check for a medical alert bracelet, necklace, or, less common, key-chain, wallet card, or kid's shoe tag. The reverse side of the tag will have basic information such as his or her name, emergency contact, and critical medical information including allergies, medications, advance medical directives, and medical conditions such as epilepsy, diabetes, or asthma.

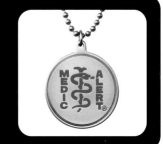

76 CALL FOR MEDEVAC

If you are far from the nearest hospital and have a serious medical emergency, you may need a helicopter medevac. When calling for help, request a helicopter rescue. Some dispatch protocols may not allow it, but if a helicopter is sent your way, here are a few important steps to follow.

STEP 1 Establish a safe landing zone. Flat, level ground 100 feet by 100 feet (30 meters by 30 meters) is ideal, clear of sand, gravel, or debris, and far from power lines, trees, poles, or other obstructions.

STEP 2 Get a fix on your position. While standing in the middle of the of the landing zone (LZ), use a GPS and note the latitude and longitude. Pass this information on to the emergency responders.

STEP 3 If the copter is landing in darkness, light up the LZ if you have the resources to do so. If you are using glow sticks, small strobes, or other portable light sources, be sure that you anchor them to the ground securely.

STEP 4 Follow these safety tips when the rescue arrives: Shield your eyes from rotor wash during landing and takeoff, do not approach the helicopter while the blades are turning, and approach it from the side only—never walk around the tail rotor.

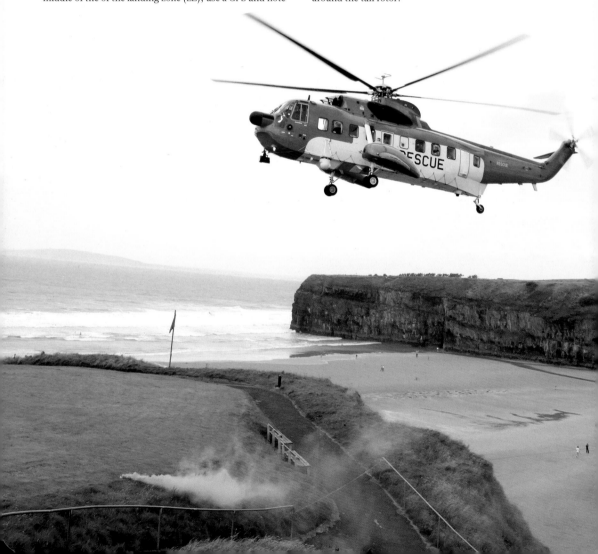

77 OPEN AN AIRWAY

The first things that you need to check when assessing an injured person are the ABCs: airway, breathing, and circulation. It's important to also do the ABCs in this order. Obviously, if you focus on stopping bleeding on a patient that isn't breathing, you're not going to have a patient for very long.

The first step to evaluate if someone has a blocked airway is to look, listen and feel for any signs of breathing. If the victim is not breathing, something

may be blocking his or her airway, in an unconscious person the most common obstruction is the tongue. To reopen the victim's airway, perform a simple head tilt/chin lift maneuver.

With the victim lying flat on his or back, place your hand on the forehead and your other hand under the tip of the chin. Gently tilt the victim's head backward. The weight of the tongue will force it to shift away from the back of the throat, opening the airway.

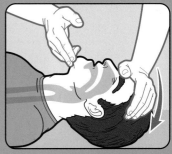

If the person is still not breathing on his or her own after the airway has been cleared, then you will have to provide rescue breathing.

78 BREATHE FOR THEM

With the victim's airway clear of any obstructions, support the chin to keep it lifted up and the head tilted back. Pinch the nose with your fingertips and place your mouth over the victim's, creating a tight seal. If available, a pocket mask (see item 67) will protect you and the victim from communicable diseases. Give two full breaths. Between each breath listen to confirm that air is escaping and watch the chest fall as the victim exhales.

Do not use excessive force when exhaling into the person's mouth, as this may force air into the stomach, causing them to vomit. If this happens, turn the person's head to the side, and clear away any obstructions from the mouth before continuing.

If the victim remains unresponsive, without any breathing, coughing, or moving, then begin CPR (see item 85).

79 CONTROL BLEEDING

After you've bandaged an injury, if blood is soaking through the bandage, you'll need to take additional action to control the bleeding. Remember to wear medical gloves if you're the one going hands-on with the patient. Don't remove the soaked bandages; add more on top of the existing ones and apply direct pressure firmly. This constricts blood vessels manually, helping to stem the excessive bleeding. If they are alert enough to do so, a patient can apply pressure directly to his or her own wound. If blood starts to show through the fresh layer of gauze, it's time to use pressure points.

80 PUT ON THE PRESSURE

In situations where direct pressure is not effective in stopping the bleeding, use the appropriate pressure point to constrict the major artery that feeds the injury. This is usually performed at a place where a pulse can be found. If this proves to be ineffective, it's time to apply a tourniquet.

AREA BLEEDING	PRESSURE POINT	LOCATION
ARM INJURIES	Brachial artery	Inner arm between shoulder and elbow
HAND INJURIES	Radial artery	Inside of wrist
LEG INJURIES	Femoral artery	Groin area along the "bikini line"
LOWER-LEG INJURIES	Popliteal artery	Behind the knee

81 USE A TOURNIQUET PROPERLY

In the event of severe bleeding, when all other methods to control it have failed, a tourniquet is a device of last resort. It can prevent someone from bleeding to death from a limb injury, although it runs the risk of damaging the limb or losing it entirely in some cases—usually only after several hours. But if you need to use a tourniquet, it can literally be a lifesaver.

STEP 1 If you can, call 911 to get medical help. Expose the bleeding injury, while keeping yourself protected with medical gloves if possible.

STEP 2 Wrap the tourniquet band around the victim's limb a couple of inches above the bleeding site. Pull the tourniquet tight so that the band cinches down against the limb very firmly, then fasten the band against itself to keep it secure. Never apply a tourniquet to a joint or around the patient's neck.

STEP 3 Twist the winding rod to continue tightening the band, until bright red bleeding has stopped and the pulse below the wound has ceased.

STEP 4 Secure the winding rod in place so that it does not come loose. Check for any bleeding or a pulse below where the tourniquet has been applied. If bleeding or pulse continues, you may need to tighten the band further or apply a second tourniquet.

STEP 5 Record the time that the tourniquet was applied so that medical professionals can properly treat the injury.

STEP 6 Assess the victim for shock (see item 100), and transport the victim to appropriate medical care as soon as possible.

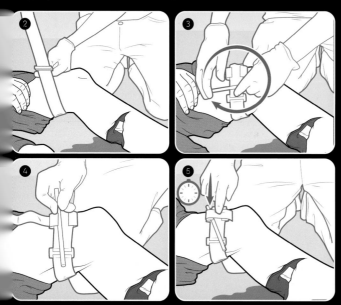

82 RIG A TOURNIQUET

If you need to help keep an injured victim from bleeding out but do not have a proper medical tourniquet, there are still plenty of good options available for you.

PICK YOUR EQUIPMENT The cinching band of a tourniquet can be made from virtually any manner of broad, flexible, sturdy substance: a leather belt or a rolled-up shirt, the rubber inner tube from a bicycle tire, braided lengths of paracord (see item 32), and lots of others besides—just as long as the material is not so thin as to cut into the tissues and cause more bleeding. Wrap the item firmly around the limb and tie it off with an overhand knot.

TWIST IT TIGHT You can use any sturdy object about the length of your forearm to apply torsion without breaking—a long sturdy stick; a wooden kitchen spoon or plastic ladle; a metal rebar, wrench, or screwdriver; and more. Place it against the cinching band that you've made and tie it in place with a square knot (see item 33). Twist it until the bleeding stops, and then secure it from unwinding with another length or cord, strip of cloth, or similar material.

GET HELP SOON Again, record the time that the tourniquet was applied, and get the victim to professional medical care as soon as you can. You've saved a life— and now you may be able to save a limb as well.

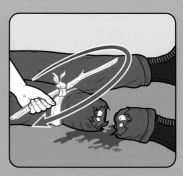

83 HELP SOMEONE WHO HAS BEEN IMPALED

While it's not a very common injury, knowing how to handle someone who has been impaled can help save their life. The Possible causes of impaling can include falling onto a sharp object such as rebar or a fence post, or trauma from high-speed accidents that involve cars, trains, or even bicycles.

STEP 1 Do not try to remove the object. Doing so could result in additional tissue damage, rapid blood loss or, if impaled in the chest, a sucking chest wound. Instead stabilize the object so that it doesn't move while the victim is moved or transported.

STEP 2 If in a remote setting where you need to move the victim without the help of emergency responders, consider cutting the object a few inches away from the injury to help make movement easier. This is usually limited to slender items such as an arrow.

STEP 3 Bandage the wound to stop bleeding and to further stabilize the object. Transport the person to a hospital only if an ambulance or helicopter isn't available to respond to the accident.

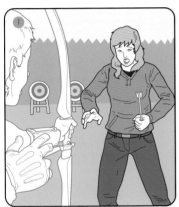
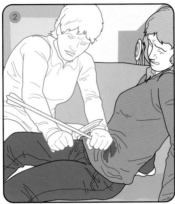
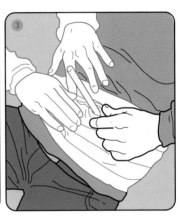

84 DEAL WITH A GUNSHOT WOUND

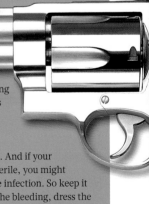

The severity of gunshot wounds varies due to a number of factors, including where the victim is hit, the caliber of the weapon, and the type of bullet used. Unless you're in the most dire circumstances in a remote location without hope for rescue, this is not the time to try your hand at any invasive procedures. Get some help—but while you're waiting for assistance to arrive there are things you can do to help stabilize the unlucky soul who has been shot.

First check the victim's ABCs (see item 77). If they are not breathing or don't have a pulse, start CPR (see item 85). If they are breathing and have a pulse, it's time to control the bleeding. Look for both entrance and exit wounds, and bandage each of them, starting with the most severe one first. If you only find an entrance wound, the bullet is still in the body, leave it alone even if you happen to feel it underneath the skin. If you're dealing with a shotgun injury, there will be numerous individual wounds to treat. There is really nothing to be gained by plucking out the shot, since disturbing the projectiles might cause more serious bleeding or other damage. And if your tools aren't sterile, you might also introduce infection. So keep it simple: Stop the bleeding, dress the wound, and let the professionals remove the bullets or shot once the victim is safely at the hospital.

85 ADMINISTER CPR

If you're preparing for emergencies, you should get trained in CPR—but even without it, you can still help.

STEP 1 Call 911 or other medical help.

STEP 2 Place the heel of your hand on the victim's sternum, with your other hand on top.

STEP 3 Lock your elbows and use your body weight to compress the chest about 2 inches (5 cm), at 100-120 compressions per minute.

STEP 4 If you're trained in CPR, after giving 30 compressions, gently tilt the victim's head back to open up their airway, and pinch their nostrils shut before delivering two breaths. Repeat steps 2-4 until help arrives or the victim recovers.

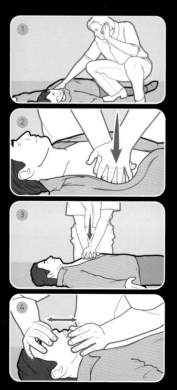

86 USE AN AED

Automatic external defibrillators, if used within the first 3-5 minutes of a cardiac arrest, can greatly improve the victim's chance of survival, from about 5 percent to 70 percent or even higher. Better yet, AEDs are designed to be used by virtually anyone, even without any experience or training. However, an AED will automatically analyze the heart's rhythm and, if necessary, give a shock to the victim in an attempt to restore the proper rhythm. AEDs will not shock patients who don't need it.

STEP 1 If you see someone collapse, immediately call 911. If there are other people on scene instruct one of them to call 911 and another to get the AED.

STEP 2 Determine whether the victim is breathing. If so, you know that they have a pulse. If the victim is not breathing, begin CPR.

STEP 3 After the AED arrives, ask a bystander to take over CPR while you apply the electrode pads that are part of the AED to the patient's bare chest. Instructions will be printed on the package or the AED for doing so. Continuous CPR is important to help save the patient. Continue CPR unless the AED is analyzing or shocking the victim.

STEP 4 Turn on the AED. Follow the visual and voice prompts of the AED to operate it correctly.

STEP 5 If advised, press the "shock" button and continue following the AED's instructions. If no shock is advised, then continue CPR until help arrives.

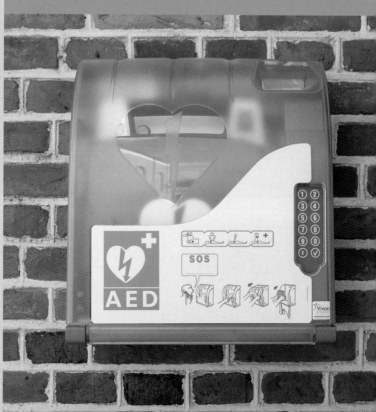

87 HELP A CHOKING VICTIM

Someone who's truly choking cannot breathe or speak. They might grab at their throat, but you must recognize the situation and act quickly.

Stand behind the victim and put your arms around their waist, with one fist below the ribs and above the navel, and your other hand covering your fist [A]. Pull up and into the victim's abdomen, pressing firmly with both hands. Repeat this motion until their airway is cleared.

If you can't reach around the person or they pass out, lay the victim on their back and perform the maneuver while straddling the legs or hips [B].

If you're dealing with a very small child or infant who is choking, cradle them in one arm and compress their chest with your fingertips five times [C], alternating this with turning them over and applying five firm slaps to the midback until the airway is cleared.

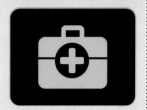
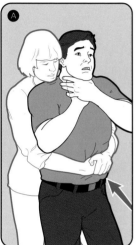

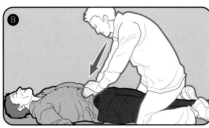

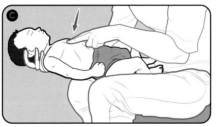

88 SAVE YOURSELF

If you're unlucky enough to choke on something while alone, you can still save yourself using a technique similar to the Heimlich. Make a fist and put your thumb below your rib cage, just above the navel. Grab your fist with your other hand, and press it into your abdomen with quick upward movements. If this doesn't work, you can also use the edge of a table, chair, or railing. Quickly and repeatedly thrust your upper abdomen against the edge. Continue until the object is dislodged and you can breathe again.

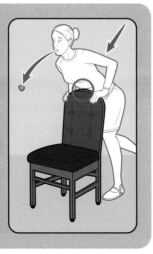

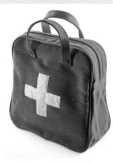

89 KNOW INJURY TYPES

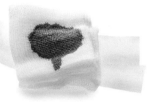

Wounds are normally categorized by specific terms that describe their characteristics to medical professionals, and understanding these will allow you to make better first-aid decisions and also communicate to emergency responders.

NAME	DESCRIPTION	CAUSE
INCISION	Clean-cut wound as if sliced by a knife	Blades, sharp edges, broken glass
LACERATION	Jagged-edged wound more resembling a tear than a slice; may have multiple branches	Object with broken or serrated edge, or blow from a blunt object
PUNCTURE	Single penetration point; may look small but can extend deep into body, causing severe bleeding or organ injuries; object sometimes remains impaled in wound	Knife or sharp object, bullet wound
ABRASION	Superficial scrape or scratch, usually affecting only skin surface layers	Result of a fall or sliding on a rough surface, often suffered by bicyclists or motorcyclists
CONTUSION	Bruising from capillaries damaged under the skin, causing swelling and discoloration; may be a sign of more serious injuries elsewhere	Blunt objects
AVULSION	Laceration with a flap of tissue mostly torn from the body; difficult to treat due to the nature of injury	Animal bites, motor vehicle collisions
AMPUTATION	Complete loss of a limb, usually with serious arterial bleeding; limbs can be reattached if carefully cooled and transported to the hospital	Industrial accidents, auto accidents, or other trauma that separates a limb from the body

90 SPOT AN INFECTION

Cleansing an injury before bandaging reduces the risk of contamination, but if it becomes infected, spotting it early can help avoid serious complications. Infection symptoms may include increased pain, swelling, redness, or warmth around the injury. There may be red streaks in the skin or pus in the wound, and the patient may have chills or fever.

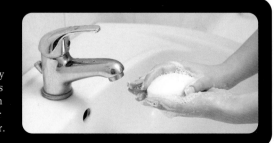

91 BANDAGE A WOUND

In the area between "this just needs a small Band-Aid" and "I'm going to need stitches" are basic wounds that can be treated as follows.

STEP 1 Wash the wound thoroughly to remove all dirt and debris; soap and water work great. Hydrogen peroxide or alcohol-based products are not recommended because of the discomfort and delay in healing.

STEP 2 Use direct pressure and elevation to control bleeding.

STEP 3 Cover the wound with a sterile dressing or bandage. If bleeding soaks through, stack more bandages over it (don't remove the dressing). Cover up with gauze, Kerlex, or Coban to secure the dressing.

STEP 4 Take an over-the-counter pain medicine if needed, such as ibuprofen or acetaminophen.

STEP 5 If there is bruising or swelling, apply ice or a cold pack for 20 minutes. Wrap this in a towel or cloth to avoid causing frostbite.

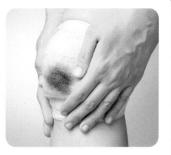

STEP 6 Keep the wound clean and dry until it is healed, which may be a number of days, or even longer depending on severity.

STEP 7 Rest the affected area and avoid intense activity.

92 SUPERGLUE IT

Dermabond is a type of adhesive that can be used instead of sutures to close a wound. It's similar to, but not exactly the same as superglue. It's important to note that superglue isn't actually approved for medical use, but in an emergency or disaster, you must decide what's the best option for you. It's equally important to remember that if you're going to use this method to close a wound that it must be thoroughly and properly cleaned first to avoid infection.

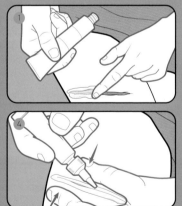
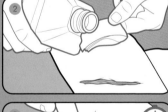
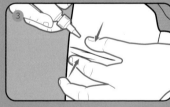
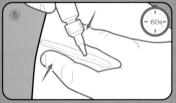
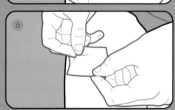

STEP 1 Apply topical anesthetic if available and if needed.

STEP 2 Clean and prepare wound with antiseptic. Dry the surrounding skin.

STEP 3 Manually close the wound with your fingers, and open the superglue.

STEP 4 Gently apply the adhesive to the surface of the laceration. Avoid allowing any adhesive into the wound.

STEP 5 Apply three layers of adhesive, while holding the wound together with fingers for at least 60 seconds after the final application.

STEP 6 Apply a dressing only after the superglue has completely dried. The injury should not be scrubbed, soaked, or picked until the adhesive naturally peels off in five to 10 days.

93 HANDLE A HEART ATTACK

A myocardial infarction, or heart attack, occurs when blood flow stops to part of the heart, causing damage to the heart muscle. A heart attack may result in irregular heartbeat, heart failure, or cardiac arrest. Common causes include lifestyle choices such as smoking; diseases such as diabetes, high blood pressure, and obesity; and genetic family history.

Some heart attacks are sudden and intense but most of them start out in a less unnerving way, with mild pain or discomfort. Sometimes people affected aren't sure what's wrong and wait before getting help.

The most common symptom is chest pain or discomfort, which may reach to the shoulder, arm, back, neck, or jaw. It is often in the center or left side of the chest, lasting for more than a few minutes, sometimes feeling like heartburn. Shortness of breath, nausea, cold sweat, or feeling faint or tired may also occur. Women are somewhat more likely than men to experience shortness of breath, nausea, vomiting, and back or jaw pain.

Since this is a potentially life-threatening condition, call 911 or get them to a hospital quickly. Also, have the patient chew an aspirin to help minimize blood clots that may be causing the heart attack.

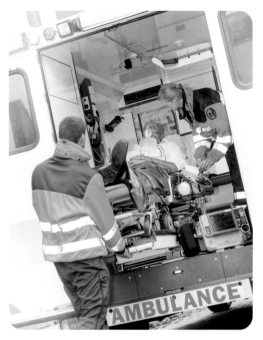

94 RECOGNIZE A STROKE

A stroke, or a cerebrovascular accident (CVA), occurs when poor blood flow to the brain results in brain damage. There are two main types: ischemic, from lack of blood flow, and hemorrhagic, caused by bleeding. Both result in part of the brain not functioning properly and both are time-critical emergencies. Strokes can happen to anyone at any time, regardless of sex or age, and of those who survive, more than two-thirds have some type of permanent disability. Minutes can make a difference, so recognizing symptoms of a stroke is the key to preventing death or disability.

If you think someone is having a stroke, ask them to smile, lift their arms, and speak a short sentence. If they fail to respond normally, you should call for an ambulance or, if during a disaster no ambulances are available, transport them to a hospital immediately yourself. Remember the mnemonic FAST.

FACIAL DROOPING Is one side of their face numb or drooping? Ask them to smile. Is it uneven?

ARM WEAKNESS Is one arm weak or numb? Ask the person to raise both arms. Does one arm waver downward?

SPEECH DIFFICULTY Are they able to speak? Is their speech slurred or hard to understand? Ask them to repeat a simple sentence. Are they able to do so correctly?

TIME TO CALL 911 If someone shows any of these symptoms—even if the symptoms go away—call 911 and get help immediately. Be sure to note when the symptoms appeared.

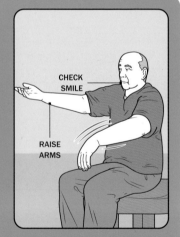

CHECK SMILE

RAISE ARMS

Other stroke symptoms include sudden trouble seeing in one or both eyes; sudden trouble with walking, dizziness, loss of coordination or balance; or sudden severe headache with no known cause. A victim may experience a combination of these symptoms, so if in doubt get them to help immediately.

95 ADDRESS AN ANXIETY ATTACK

Anxiety attacks, also called panic attacks, are episodes of intense panic or fear. They usually occur suddenly and without warning, peak within 10 minutes, and rarely last more than 30 minutes. Shortness of breath and chest pain are sometimes the most significant symptoms; the person may fear incorrectly that they are suffering a heart attack. However, since chest pain and shortness of breath are the hallmark symptoms of cardiovascular illnesses, seeking an emergency medical evaluation is still appropriate to determine the true cause.

SYMPTOMS OF ANXIETY INCLUDE:

- feeling overwhelmed, detached, or unreal
- feeling like you are losing control or going crazy
- heart palpitations or chest pain
- feeling faint, dizzy, or light-headed
- hyperventilation, trouble breathing, or sensation of choking
- hot flashes or chills (particularly in the facial or neck area)
- trembling or shaking
- nausea or stomach cramps
- numbness or tingling throughout the body
- headache or backache
- sweating
- dry mouth or difficulty swallowing

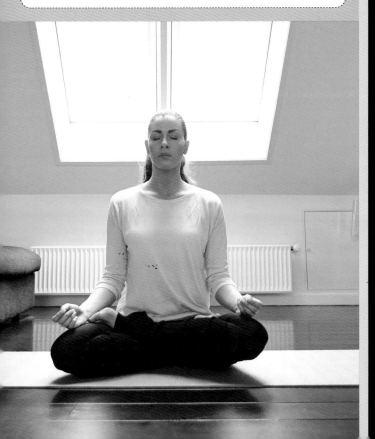

96 HELP THEM CALM DOWN

Being there for somebody who is experiencing an anxiety attack can really make a big difference to their well-being. Here are some ways to help calm someone under these circumstances.

The person will probably have an overwhelming desire to leave where they are; help them get somewhere quiet and secure. Try to reassure the person repeatedly by letting them know that you're going to help and support them. If you are able to get them into a safe space, reassure them that they are safe.

If the person is having an anxiety attack, get their permission before making physical contact. In some cases, touching without asking can increase the panic and make the situation worse.

Ask the victim what will help them. Sometimes people will know what will help, but may need your assistance to initiate the activity. Accept that their fear is very real to them, and that if you minimize or dismiss the fear in any way you can make the panic attack worse. Let them talk it out or process their experience, for example, by asking them questions in a calm, neutral way. Listen supportively and accept whatever answer is given.

Help the victim to control their breathing by taking slow, deliberate breaths. Ask them to inhale and exhale on your count. Start off by counting out loud, encouraging the victim to inhale for two seconds and then out for another two. After that, gradually increase the count until they have slowed their breathing.

Some panic attacks can also be accompanied by sensations of warmth, commonly around the neck and face. A cool, damp cloth can help minimize this sensation and calm the victim. Stay with the person until they have recovered from the attack.

97 HELP A SEIZURE VICTIM

Seizures result from abnormal electrical activity in the brain caused by fever, injury, stroke, brain tumors, or certain medications. Seizures occurring on a regular basis are a condition called epilepsy. There are several types of seizures, but tonic-clonic seizures are one of the most significant. The person may go rigid, fall down, and then convulse for a minute or two. Their breathing may also be affected and they may go pale or blue, particularly around the mouth; they may also lose bladder or bowel control.

This can be frightening to see, but isn't often a medical emergency. Once the convulsions have ended, the person usually recovers slowly. They may appear "spaced out" or unable to easily answer questions for some time after the seizure ends.

If possible, ease the seizing person to the floor. Protect them from injury by moving any hard or sharp objects and put a soft, flat item, such as a pillow, under their head. Make note of how long the seizures last; report the information to medical responders. Place the victim in the recovery position (see item 99) once the seizure is over, and stay with them until recovery is complete. Be calmly reassuring throughout. Do not restrain the person or try to move them unless they are in danger, and do not place anything in their mouth or give them anything to eat or drink until they are fully recovered.

Call an ambulance if the seizure lasts more than a few minutes or they have another seizure without regaining consciousness; if they are injured, have trouble breathing, or become aggressive after the seizure; or if they have other health conditions such as diabetes, heart disease, or are pregnant.

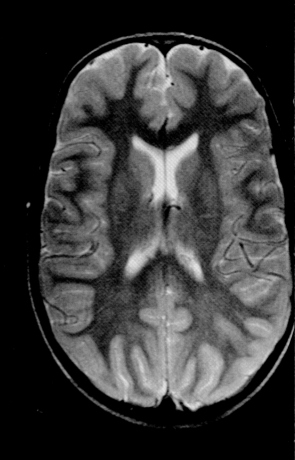

98 PROTECT A PATIENT'S SPINE

The bones of the neck, referred to as the cervical vertebrae or c-spine, may be fractured or displaced if the neck has been twisted, compressed, or hyper-extended due to trauma. This can lead to severing or compression of their spinal cord, resulting in permanent nerve damage and paralysis. Assume someone has c-spine injury if they have neck pain after serious injury such as vehicle or bicycle accidents, falls, sport injuries, or assaults.

If the victim is awake, tell them to keep still and let them know you're going to help them by immobilizing their neck. Kneel above their head, and place both hands on either side of the victim's head to steady it. Hold onto their head gently but firmly to prevent movement. Any movement of the cervical spine may make a c-spine injury worse. Until medical help gets there, only release the victim's head to help with their airway, breathing or circulation, or if it becomes unsafe to remain at the scene.

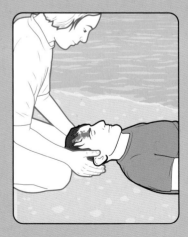

99 HELP A VICTIM RECOVER

If a sick or injured person is unconscious but is breathing and has no other life-threatening conditions or spinal injuries, they should be placed in the recovery position. Putting someone in the recovery position will ensure their airway remains clear and open. It also prevents vomit or other body fluids to be inhaled or cause choking, both of which can be life threatening.

STEP 1 Kneel on the floor on one side of the person.

STEP 2 Place the arm nearest you at a right angle to their body with their hand upwards above their head.

STEP 3 Tuck the victim's other hand under the side of their head, so that the back of their hand is touching their cheek.

STEP 4 Bend and lift the knee farthest from you to a right angle.

STEP 5 Carefully roll the person towards you onto their side by pulling on the bent knee and their shoulder.

STEP 6 Once on their side, tuck the bent knee up towards their hips to keep them stable on their side.

STEP 7 Open the person's airway by doing a head tilt/chin lift maneuver (see item 77) by gently tilting their head back and lifting their chin. Check that nothing is blocking their airway. Stay with the person and monitor their breathing and pulse until help arrives. Reassure the patient while you wait.

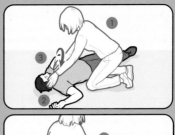
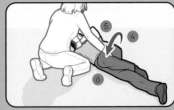
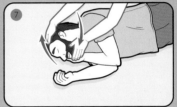
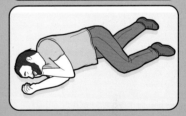

100 TREAT FOR SHOCK

In shock, the body's organs and tissues are not receiving an adequate flow of blood. This is a common condition after an accident and can result in serious damage or even death. Symptoms can include anxiety, restlessness, or nervousness; confusion or even loss of awareness; rapid pulse; rapid, shallow breathing; pale, cool, sweaty skin; blotchy or bluish skin (especially around the mouth and lips); dilated pupils that are slow to respond to light; thirst; and nausea or vomiting.

It's best to assume that all parties who have been injured in an accident will develop shock; proactively treat them before symptoms develop. Early treatment can reduce the severity of the shock, and help save a life.

STEP 1 Have the person lie down, and their head flat on the ground. Treat any injuries, such as bleeding.

STEP 2 Elevate the victim's feet slightly.

STEP 3 Loosen restrictive clothing and belts to help them breathe more easily.

STEP 4 Keep them warm with blankets or coats.

STEP 5 Calmly talk and reassure the person until help arrives. Do not give them anything to eat or drink.

101 RECOGNIZE A HAIRLINE FRACTURE

A hairline fracture is the medical term for a crack in the bone, rather than a full break. However, should the crack worsen or break entirely, things could get complicated; you might even need surgery to correct the problem.

Hairline fractures are tricky because they can seem more like a strain or sprain than a fracture, which, while painful, may not be swollen, bruised, or deformed and is likely to have more normal function. It's only when the pain doesn't decrease after about three or four days that some people will suspect that something else is wrong. If you have an injury that remains painful after several days, get it evaluated. If you're in a disaster situation where medical attention isn't easily accessible, it's best to assume that it's broken and splint the injury site to protect it.

102 STABILIZE A FRACTURE

Fortunately, a fracture is often a stable injury. Getting to a hospital is always the best recourse, but if medical attention isn't readily available, splinting and, if it's needed, setting a bone can help you manage the pain and discomfort. In fact, a closed reduction might be the only way to save the arm or leg. Here's how you can do it.

ASSESS THE INJURY A fracture usually won't need any setting, but it might if the bone has broken clean across or diagonally, or is broken in multiple fragments that are jamming into one another. If the bone is protruding from the skin, don't try to set it. Just splint it in place and cover it with a moist dressing.

CHECK CIRCULATION Press on the skin past the fracture site. The skin should turn white and then change back to pink quickly. Pale or bluish skin, a lack of a pulse in the limb, numbness, or tingling might indicate a loss of proper circulation.

REDUCE THE FRACTURE To decrease swelling, pain, and damage to the tissues caused by any lack of circulation, realign the limb into a normal position by slowly and carefully pulling in opposite directions on both sides of the break. This is usually easiest with two people.

SPLINT THE LIMB Use a splint to keep the break stable and in place.

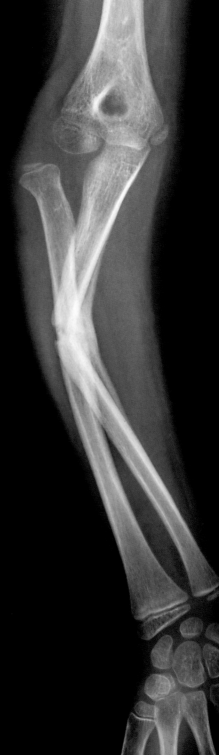

103 SLING AN INJURED ARM

A sling is the easiest way to comfortably stabilize an arm injury such as a fracture, a severe sprain, or even an especially deep laceration. Knowing how to improvise a sling is useful—especially since you'll want to do so regardless if you're on your way to the hospital or if you're forced to wait until medical care becomes available.

STEP 1 Start with a cloth about 3 feet by 3 feet (1 meter by 1 meter). Lay the cloth out flat, and then fold it once diagonally to make a triangle. (Your first aid kit should contain at least two cloth slings.)

STEP 2 Slip the injured arm into the fold, and bring both ends up around the neck, slanting the forearm upward very slightly.

STEP 3 Tie the corners in a knot, including the one near the elbow to create a pocket for it to rest in. This will naturally allow the forearm to stay in the sling easily.

STEP 4 Use your second sling (if improvising, use a belt) to immobilize the arm against the body. Wrap it around the chest above the forearm and above the problematic zone. Cinch it closed but not too tightly, as circulation is key.

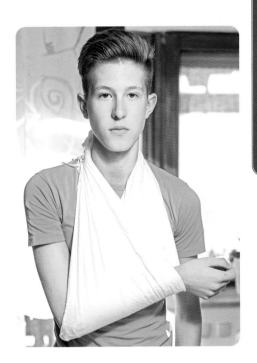

104 SPLINT A LIMB

If someone injures a limb, especially at the joint, immobilization is key to stabilize the injury. Craft a splint with padding (such as some cloth or a T-shirt), tape, cardboard and other flexible material to support the area.

STEP 1 Stop any bleeding using direct pressure or a tourniquet if needed (see item 81).

STEP 2 Check for a pulse below the injury. The inside of the wrist and the top of the foot are common places to check. Remember to use your fingers and not your thumb to check for a pulse (your thumb has a pulse and you might mistake it for that of your patient).

STEP 3 Slide the cardboard or other splint material beneath the limb, and pad it for comfort and stability.

STEP 4 Fold the splint around the limb, securing it with tape, paracord, or other material. The splint should be just tight enough to prevent the limb from shifting but not so tight that it impedes circulation. Secure the splint both above and below the injury for added stability.

STEP 5 Check for a pulse below the injury again. Recheck every 20 minutes or so to make sure circulation isn't lost. If the patient complains of numbness or tingling, or you can't find a pulse, loosen the splint slightly.

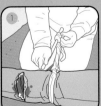 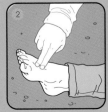 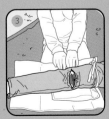 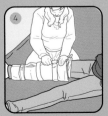 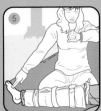

105 IDENTIFY AND TREAT BURNS

Skin is the body's largest organ and is made of layers of varying thicknesses. The severity of a burn depends on how deeply into these layers it penetrates, and the treatment varies for each type of burn. Regardless of severity, remove jewelry, belts, and any other restrictive clothing, especially from around the burned areas, as those tissues may rapidly become swollen.

1ST DEGREE Also known as superficial burns, these can be caused by almost anything from hot liquids to excess sun exposure. They heal on their own, but you should remove any constraining jewelry or clothing and apply a cool compress or aloe vera gel. Taking anti-inflammatory drugs may also hasten healing and improve comfort.

2ND DEGREE Flame flashes, boiling liquids, and hot metals cause this burn, which usually penetrates to the skin's second layer. Blisters will occur, and it will take more than a few days to heal. Flood the site with cool water and trim away any loose skin (but leave blisters intact to prevent infection). Apply burn gel and change nonadhesive dressings daily. If the burn area is greater than 3 inches (7.5 cm) in diameter, or if it is on the victim's face, hands, feet, groin, or buttocks, visit an emergency room for care if possible.

3RD DEGREE Full-thickness burns are very severe, reaching through all three layers of the skin. Treat the victim for shock and transport them to a hospital. Cover the burns loosely with a sterile burn sheet or use the cleanest cloth available. Do not moisten the bandage, as that can cause hypothermia. Skin grafts and extensive medical care will be required.

4TH DEGREE This burn will damage structures below the skin, such as tendons, muscles, and bones. These burns are very serious and potentially life-threatening, and because this type of burn destroys nerves, the victim may not complain significantly about pain or sensation. Permanent disability and death are both serious possibilities, so it's critical to evacuate the victim to a medical facility immediately. As with third-degree burns, cover with a dry sterile burn dressing.

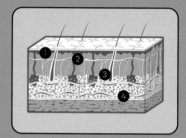

106 CARE FOR CHEMICAL BURNS

One of the biggest challenges for dealing with chemical burns is the sheer variety of chemicals and knowing the appropriate response for each. If you do happen to know exactly what chemical is responsible, check the original packaging for first aid instructions. You can also look up the substance's Material Safety Data Sheet (MSDS), which has additional technical information for fire fighting, protective equipment, and containment and cleanup safety. If you're not entirely certain as to the nature of the substance causing the burn, follow these general guidelines.

STEP 1 Remove the chemical causing the burn carefully. For dry chemicals, brush off any remaining material. Wear gloves or use a towel or a brush rather than using your hands.

STEP 2 Remove contaminated clothing and jewelry.

STEP 3 Rinse the burn immediately. Run a gentle stream of cool water over the burn for 10 or more minutes. Be sure to avoid any contaminated water splashing into the eyes of the patient.

STEP 4 Loosely apply a bandage.

STEP 5 If needed, take an over-the-counter pain reliever.

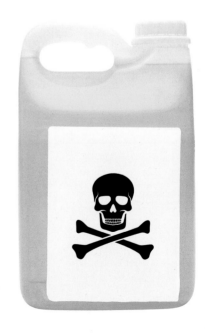

107 AVOID LIVE WIRES

If the victim is still being shocked by a source of electricity, or the risk for shock hasn't been eliminated, you have to keep yourself safe before you can help.

If the person is affected by an indoor power source, shut it off or unplug it, or cut off power at the circuit breaker or fuse box. You can also use a nonconductive object such as a wooden broom handle (if you can, stand on a wooden board, phone book, or similar dry nonconducting surface) to break the circuit. If the power source is outdoors, but no greater than residential power, the same techniques can apply.

Don't get near high-voltage wires until the power is turned off. Usually the local power company must do so. Since overhead power lines usually aren't insulated, stay at least 30 feet away if wires are jumping and sparking, or 60 feet in wet conditions. If you feel a tingling in your legs and lower body in the disaster area, you're on electrified ground; to avoid being electrocuted, hop on one foot away from the source of electricity (as both feet create a full circuit). If a power line falls on a car, instruct the passengers to stay inside until officials say it's safe.

108 HELP A SHOCKED PERSON

The harmful effects of an electrical shock depend on several factors, including the type of current, voltage, and how the current has traveled through the body. An electrical shock may cause burns, or it may leave no detectable marks. In either case, any electrical current passing through the body can result in severe internal injuries.

The effects of high voltage can include severe burns inside and outside the victim's body; seizures, confusion, or loss of consciousness; muscle pain and spasms; and difficulty breathing, heart arrhythmia, and cardiac arrest.

If someone has been shocked, call 911 or your local emergency number, especially if the source is a lightning strike or high-voltage wire. (Don't touch the injured person if he or she is still in contact with the electrical current.) Begin CPR if required, treat any burns, and treat for shock.

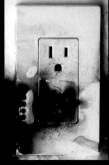

109 HANDLE HYPOTHERMIA

If you were paying attention in high school biology class, you'll remember that the ideal temperature for the human body is about 98.6 °F (37 °C). If a person's core body temperature drops below 95 °F (35 °C), you've got a case of hypothermia on your hands. Symptoms range from mild chills to coma and even death, depending on how low the core body temperature drops.

Treating hypothermia is simple and direct: Start off by making sure the person is out of danger. If the environment is cold enough to cause hypothermia in the victim, then it can put you at risk, too. Next, get the victim out of any wet clothing. You'll want to wrap them in blankets or coats and, if possible, place warm water bottles or chemical hand warmers in the armpits, groin, and stomach. A warm, sweet drink will help—just avoid the old adage about drinking warm booze; alcohol actually speeds up heat loss. Monitor them carefully and if they become confused or their face, hands, or feet show signs of frostbite, get them to a hospital.

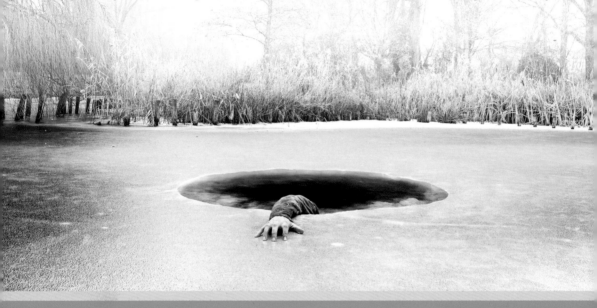

110 AVOID FROSTBITE

If you frequently find yourself outside in very cold conditions, learning to avoid frostbite is wise, given the potentially severe consequences. Frostbite prevention involves having a working knowledge of protective clothing against cold and wind.

COVER UP Wear several layers of light, loose clothing to help provide better protection than a single bulky layer of heavy clothing. Choose fabrics suited for the cold (such as fleece, polypropylene, or wool). Avoid restrictive and tight clothing.

PROTECT YOUR EXTREMITIES Wear mittens instead of gloves; if mittens have to be temporarily removed to allow use of the fingers, wear lightweight gloves under them for additional protection. Wear two pairs of socks, and cover the face and head as much as reasonably possible, especially the ears.

BE SELF-AWARE Keep hydrated, and do not drink alcohol or smoke. Avoid staying still for too long, getting wet, or any prolonged exposure to the elements; seek shelter from wind and cold whenever possible. Retreat to warmth and safety if you notice early signs of frostbite: stinging, burning, throbbing, or a prickling sensation followed by numbness.

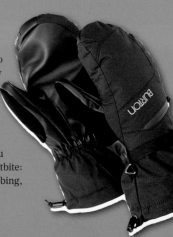

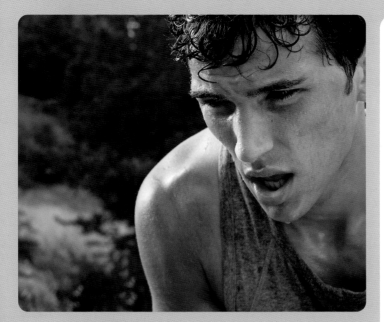

112
DEFEAT DEHYDRATION

Humans can go a while without food, but a lack of water is an entirely different story. Without a constant supply of potable water, dehydration will set in quickly, along with low energy, poor judgment, and, in extreme cases, the eventual loss of the will to survive.

You should regularly drink fluids, preferably pure water. Don't wait until you're thirsty to drink. Get used to being on a hydration schedule and stick to it, especially during disasters.

Your risk of dehydration is just as high in the cold as it is in the heat. Every breath you take releases moisture into the dry air, and when it's cold, you're probably less thirsty.

We all know that activity in the heat leads to dehydration if we don't drink enough water, but it's worse at high elevation: The air is arid and thin, so you end up breathing harder and sweating more, which in turn accelerates dehydration.

If you begin to experience signs of dehydration, drink clear fluids, including water, clear broths, or electrolyte-containing beverages such as coconut water. An excess of pure water on its own—after you've lost salts and other minerals from sweating—can be dangerous.

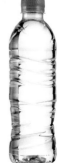

111 SURVIVE HEAT ILLNESS

There's heat, and then there's extreme heat—the kind that skyrockets your core body temperature to 104°F (40°C), making you dizzy and hot to the touch, and even rendering you unconscious. In severe circumstances, heat illness can even be fatal.

The milder of the two heat-related ailments, heat exhaustion, can occur when the body's temperature gets too high. Victims of heat exhaustion can experience dizziness, nausea, fatigue, profuse sweating, and clammy skin. Treatment is simple: Have the victim lie down in the shade, elevate their feet, and supply plenty of fluids [A].

If someone's core body temperature reaches 104°F (40°C), they will need immediate treatment for heatstroke, which can be deadly. Aside from an alarming thermometer reading, the easiest signs to identify are hot, dry skin, headache, dizziness, and even unconsciousness. To treat, elevate the victim's head and wrap them in a wet sheet [B].

Heatstroke is a life-threatening emergency and requires immediate treatment in a hospital setting, as heatstroke can damage the kidneys, brain, and heart if it goes on for too long at too high a temperature.

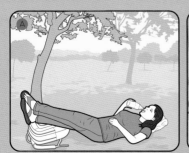

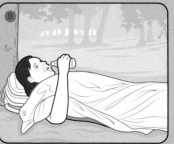

113 BEWARE COMMON POISONS

We all know it's important to keep household cleansers, detergent, and bleach away from children. The same goes for medicines—pills can look like candy to kids. But do other dangerous substances lurk in your home?

CHECK YOUR BATHROOM Beware of nail-polish remover, shampoo, and even mouthwash. Due to the ingredients or alcohol content, the majority of personal-care products can be poisonous if ingested.

CLEAR THE GARAGE Pesticides, paints, paint thinners and removers, fuels, and oil are all highly dangerous to inhale or swallow. That's pretty obvious from the smell, but other substances to watch for include antifreeze and windshield-washer fluid, which, while deadly, are brightly colored and may have a sweet taste or smell.

MAKE YOUR KITCHEN SAFE It's well known that raw or undercooked poultry or fish can be a source of foodborne illness such as salmonella. Less well known is the fact that uncooked beans also warrant caution. Nearly all varieties, especially red kidney beans, contain substances called lectins, which are broken down by cooking but, if eaten uncooked, can cause nausea, vomiting, and diarrhea.

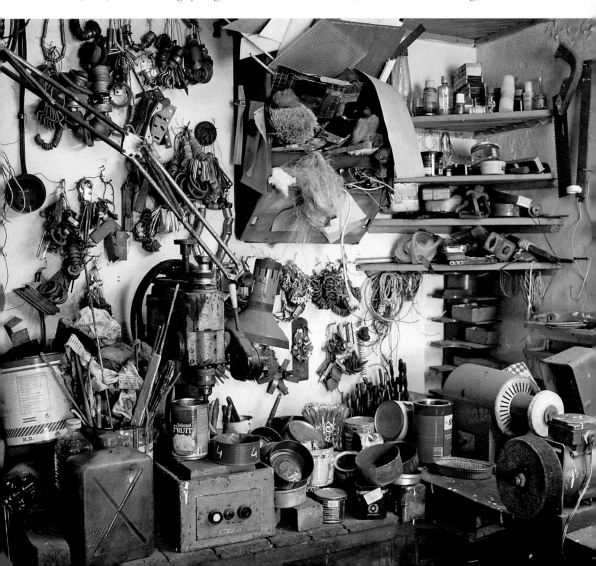

114 KNOW SIGNS OF POISONING

If you need to evaluate a child for poisoning, or if someone refuses to answer questions about what they may have ingested, as in the case of a suicidal person, you can look for these common signs.

The victim may have burns or redness around the mouth and lips, or burns, stains and odors on their body, clothing, or other objects nearby. They may also have paint, powders, or other liquids around the face and nostrils. Likewise, a strong chemical odor, such as gasoline or paint thinner, may be on their breath. Look for any empty medication bottles or scattered pills, or spilled or empty containers for chemical, paint, or household products.

The individual may show signs of nausea or begin vomiting, become drowsy or unconscious, experience difficulty breathing, or even respiratory arrest. The victim may also be agitated or restless, or seizing or twitching uncontrollably. Assume that the person is poisoned until proven otherwise, and take action on treating a poisoning victim (see item 115).

If the person has no symptoms, but you suspect poisoning, call your regional poison control center. Provide age, weight, and any information you may have about the poison, such as how much of it was ingested and how long since the person was first exposed to it. If possible, it will help to have the pill bottle or container on hand when you call.

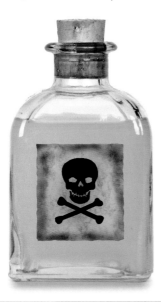

115 TREAT A POISONING VICTIM

Helping a poisoning victim can be tricky, since there's no one-size-fits-all solution. But in every case, it's vital to find out what the toxin is and seek help.

STEP 1 Call your local emergency number to request help.

STEP 2 If the poison is emitting fumes or there is a strong chemical odor in the room, move the person into fresh air.

STEP 3 Put on gloves, if available, to prevent getting contamination. Check for any remaining poisonous substance on the victim's face. If you find any, wipe it away. If the poison has spilled on the person's clothing, remove the affected clothing.

STEP 4 If the victim isn't breathing, and you have a CPR mask or face shield, and you're certified in CPR, begin rescue breathing.

STEP 5 If poison got exposed on bare skin or in the eyes, flush with lukewarm water for 20 minutes or until help arrives.

STEP 6 If the toxin is a household product, check the label for advice, or contact your local poison-control hotline. Do not induce vomiting or administer a charcoal slurry unless instructed to do so.

STEP 7 If the victim goes to the emergency room, take the pill bottle or package that contained what was ingested. That will help doctors start proper treatment immediately.

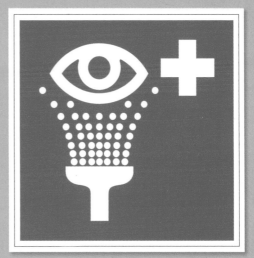

116

DON'T PANIC OVER PREGNANCY

Modern Western society tends to regard labor as a kind of emergency requiring medical intervention. In most situations, however, nothing could be farther from the truth. Women have been delivering babies for thousands of years without the benefit of modern medicine and, unless there is a complication, the delivery can safely be performed just about anywhere. If a mother-to-be is prepared and is in good health, if the location is safe, and if there are aren't any other known complications, let nature take its course and help deliver a new life into the world.

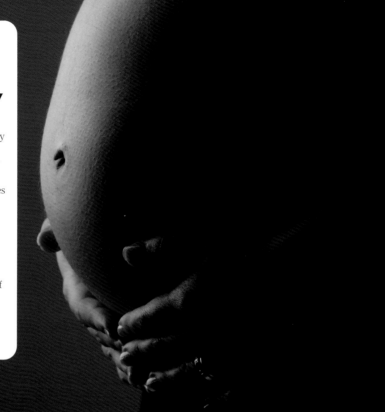

117 DEAL WITH LABOR

Labor is the first stage of the process that leads to the actual delivery of the baby. Here's what you can do to help.

STEP 1 Decide whether to transport the mother-to-be to the hospital, call an ambulance, or help deliver the baby. If labor has just started, it will usually be fine to give her a ride to the hospital if that's what she wants, or call an ambulance if she prefers. If she is late in labor, then the decision will be made for you, and you'll want to prepare for the delivery.

STEP 2 Time contractions from the beginning of one to the beginning of the next, and note how long they last. If they are 5 or more minutes apart, you have time to get the mother to the hospital if she wants to go. If the contractions are two or fewer minutes apart, then prepare for delivery. If she feels like she's going to have a bowel movement, delivery is imminent.

STEP 3 Protect the baby from possible infection by washing your hands thoroughly with soap and warm water all the

way up to your elbows. If you lack soap and water, use a hand sanitizing product or rubbing alcohol. Wear medical gloves if you have them available.

STEP 4 Prepare the birthing area. Gather several clean sheets or towels. Have the mother undress from the waist down and offer her a clean sheet or towel to cover up. Find a few pillows to help her be positioned more comfortably during delivery. Fill a clean bowl with warm water, and get a pair of scissors, a length of paracord, and a bulb syringe.

STEP 5 Help the mother stay calm. It may help if you speak to her in a low, soothing voice and work to verbally direct her breathing (or take deep, slow breaths along with her).

STEP 6 Help the mother find a comfortable position, or she may want to walk around or crouch down, especially when she has a contraction. Allow her to find her own position of comfort, which may be lying back, squatting, or on all fours.

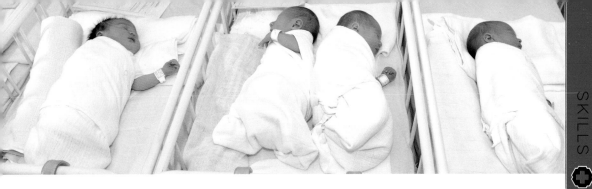

118 DELIVER A BABY

If the mother has delivered children in the past, the actual delivery can be quite fast, but if it's her first time it's normal for the process to take longer.

STEP 1 To avoid exhausting the mother, don't encourage her to push until she feels an unstoppable pressure. Eventually, the area around the vagina will bulge, and the top of the baby's head will become visible. Continue to encourage her to push gently between contractions and to take deep, slow breaths to help manage the pain.

STEP 2 Support the baby's head as it emerges, allowing it to rotate to one side. Don't pull, as this might hurt the baby.

STEP 3 Keep supporting the baby's head and neck as a shoulder will normally emerge with the next push. Deliver the other shoulder by gently lifting the body if needed.

STEP 4 The rest of the body will follow quickly. Hold the delivered baby with two hands, one supporting its neck and head. The newborn will be slippery, so dry them off with a towel and tilt their head down with the legs slightly elevated to allow any fluids to drain.

STEP 5 Ensure the baby is breathing. If it's not crying, rub the body to stimulate it. Gently suction fluids from mouth and nostrils with a bulb syringe. If the baby turns blue, perform infant CPR (see item 119).

STEP 6 If the baby is breathing, place them on the mother's chest with full-skin contact, and cover both of them with clean towels or a blanket. (The skin contact will stimulate the release of a hormone that helps to deliver the placenta.) Encourage the mother to breast feed the newborn, as it helps reduce bleeding by contracting the uterus.

STEP 7 Massage the abdomen to both assist delivery of the placenta (which can take up to an hour to occur) and help control bleeding—do not pull on the umbilical cord! Once the placenta is delivered, you can wrap it in plastic in case it is needed for inspection.

STEP 8 If an ambulance is on the way, you can wait for them to cut the cord. Otherwise, wait for the cord to stop pulsing, then tie it off in two places a few inches apart and 3 inches (7.5 cm) from the baby using some paracord. Sever the cord between the two knots with sterilized scissors.

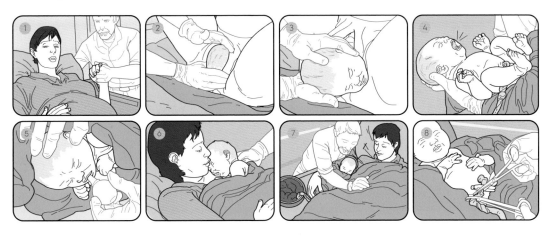

119 PERFORM INFANT CPR

If you have helped deliver a baby and they are not crying or moving, you should stimulate them by drying and warming them, rubbing their limbs or body, and checking to see if the infant's airway is clear of mucus or fluids. A newborn infant should breathe at least 30-60 times per minute, and have a pulse rate between 100 and 160. If they don't respond to any of the manual stimulation, are turning blue, or don't have a pulse, then you will need to perform infant CPR.

STEP 1 Hold the baby in one arm with the head in the palm of your hand, or lay them down on a flat, padded surface; keep their head level, not tucked or hyperextended.

STEP 2 Start by delivering 30 chest compressions at a rate of 100-120 per minute by placing the tips of two or three of fingers in the middle of the infant's chest, and apply compression to a depth of about 1.5 inches (4 cm).

STEP 3 Open the airway using a head tilt/chin lift, but do not tilt the head too far back. Deliver two rescue breaths by covering their mouth and nose with your mouth and giving just a small puff of air each time.

STEP 4 After two minutes, check for a pulse on the brachial artery, located inside the upper arm. Briefly pause to call for an ambulance at this time.

STEP 5 Continue delivering compressing and breaths at a ratio of 30:2.

STEP 6 After two minutes, check for a pulse on the brachial artery inside the upper arm. Repeat steps 5 and 6 until emergency responders arrive, obvious signs of life return, you become too exhausted to continue, or if the scene becomes unsafe.

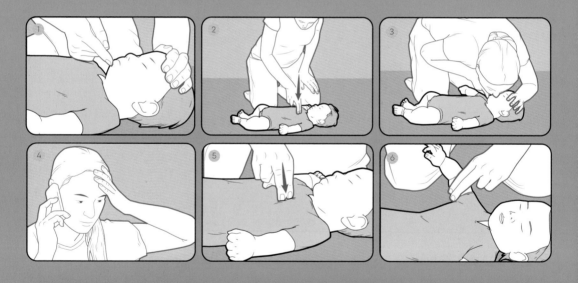

120 HAVE A HELPER

Ideally, you will have someone else with you if you are delivering a baby for all kinds of reasons. One vital reason is that they can assist you in the unlikely event that you need to give CPR. Here's how. With the infant lying on a pad, one person can support the head and deliver rescue breaths. The second will deliver chest compressions by encircling the newborn's torso with both hands, using his or her thumbs side by side in the middle of the chest instead of two fingertips. The proper compression-to-breath ratio for two-person CPR is 30:2. To maintain effective CPR for as long as possible, switch positions after 2 minutes while checking for a pulse.

121 BE A HELPFUL PARENT

If you're a parent with a child who's sick or otherwise in need of medical help, you can still make things easier even if you're not a medical professional yourself.

HOLD YOUR BABY Sit your child on your lap. It will make them more comfortable while interacting with a stranger.

GIVE COMFORT Reassure your child and keep repeating calming words to keep them calm throughout the experience.

KEEP CALM By remaining calm yourself you'll help keep your child calm.

BE AN ADVOCATE If the people are not treating your child appropriately, advocate for your child's needs.

AID WITH INFORMATION Be ready to provide details about your child's medical history if needed.

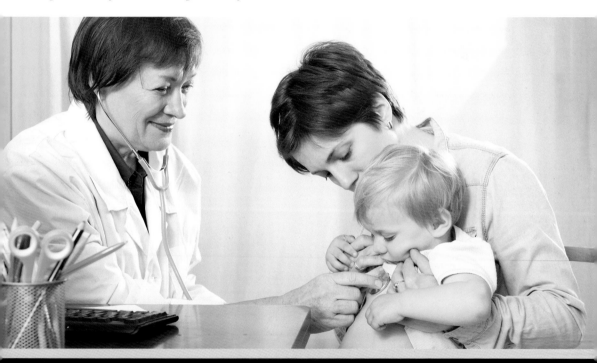

122 BE PATIENT WITH LITTLE PATIENTS

Sick children make anxious parents and can often even make medical professionals nervous. Since they can't always answer questions or say what's bothering them with any clarity, it's frequently hard for both parents and paramedics to figure out what's bothering them. If you're trying to help a child, you can help them much more easily if you work with them.

Sit or crouch down next to the child so you're closer to their height. If you speak with a quiet, calm, and confident voice, you'll be able to easier establish a rapport with the child and make it easier to help them.

Relate to the child and be empathetic. Explain to them

what you are doing, step by step, so they are not surprised by what's happening. Assume the child understand what you're saying. You can even find a toy or stuffed animal to "treat" first before you start treating the child, so that they may know what to expect.

Make the space in which you're caring for the child as comfortable as possible. If it's loud, dark, or cold, move to someplace quieter, with better light, or someplace warmer. Smells, animals, and too many people surrounding a young patient are also factors to consider. Remove anything that might be stressful or upsetting to the child if possible.

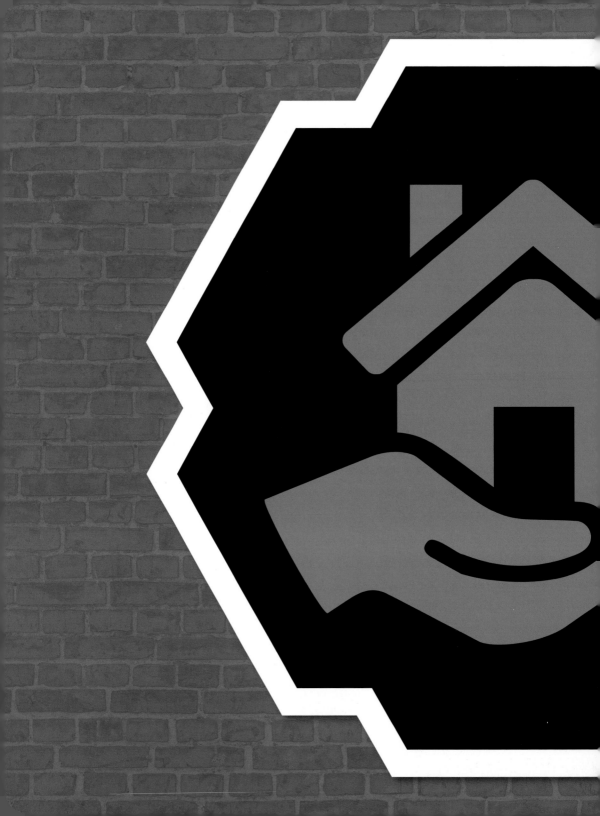

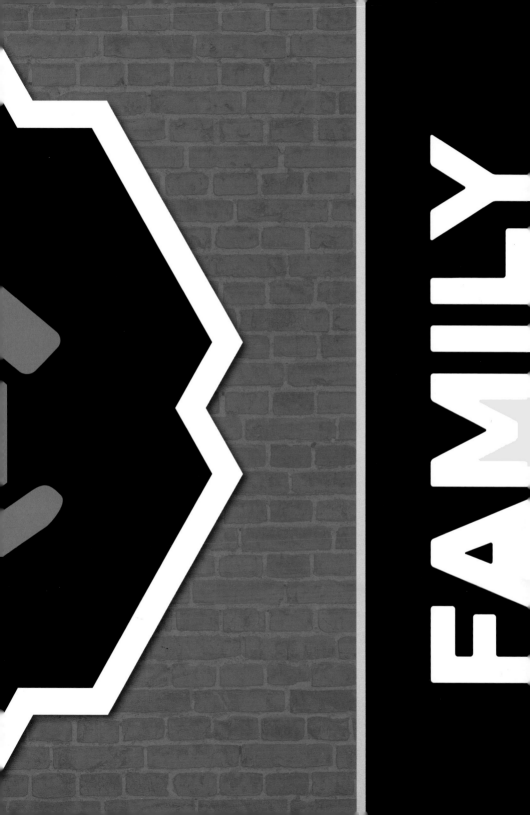

FAMILY

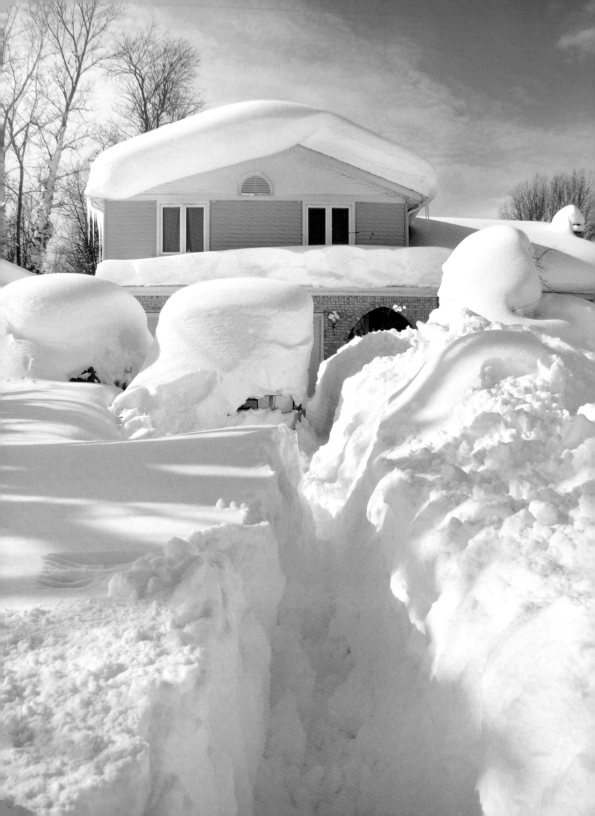

SOMETIMES BEING PREPARED MAKES MODERN-DAY HASSLES OR MINOR EMERGENCIES MUCH MORE BEARABLE AND SATISFYING TO OVERCOME. WE WERE IN AN AREA WITH NO CELL PHONE COVERAGE, HIGHWAY ADVISORY SIGNS,

department of transportation AM radio traffic information, or any kind of local FM radio signal for that matter. Fortunately, I have two-way radio equipment installed in my 4x4 SUV, so I was able to talk to other HAM radio operators and monitor the Highway Patrol frequencies to find out just how bad the situation was. With this information, we were able to calculate an alternative route, squeeze off the freeway, all while others were stuck for 12 hours or more.

Most emergencies you'll face in life won't be large-scale disasters, but that doesn't mean they're not serious. This section will give you tools and strategies to deal with crises involving your home, your family, your pets, and other aspects of everyday life from being stuck in an elevator to foiling pickpockets to facing down aggressive dogs to coping with traffic accidents. Want to ensure your family's safety? Learn how to make an emergency plan, cope with intruders and prevent house fires. Interested in gear? Figure out what kind of everyday carry (EDC) kit you need and the type of communications gear you want to invest in. Worried about your children? Read about how to handle missing kids, childproof your home, and help kids prepare in various age-appropriate ways for disasters.

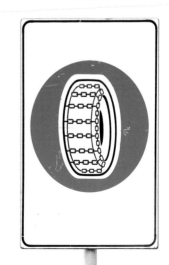

123 GRAB YOUR GO BAG

A go bag is a collection of items that you would need to survive if you had to flee your home with no guarantee of shelter, food, or water during an emergency. Think of it as your survival insurance policy. There may not be one universally agreed-upon set of equipment but, with a good core set of items, you can put together a go bag suited for a wide variety of situations.

It's best to use a backpack so that you can easily carry your gear. Fill it up with the minimum following things, with items sealed in zip-top bags to keep them organized and prevent them getting wet.

- Shelter items like a small tent and sleeping bag (if you want to go ultraminimalist, pack a tarp and a space blanket)
- Drinking water and purification equipment
- High-calorie, no-cook foods such as protein bars, peanut butter, trail mix, etc.
- First-aid, sanitation, and hygiene supplies
- Several fire-starting options
- A small pot for boiling water or cooking
- Basic tools such as a knife, duct tape, and paracord
- Extra clothes appropriate for all seasons
- Flashlight with extra batteries
- Cash and a spare debit card
- A thumb drive with a backup of important documents: bank info, insurance documents, wills, and personal items such as family photos or videos

Stash your main go bag safe and ready to go in a secure location, with smaller versions in your car and office. It's also a good idea for you to have everyday carry (EDC) items—survival essentials that you can carry in your pocket or purse.

HOME GO BAG

Emergency rations (MREs, food bars, etc) · Bottled water · Tent & tarp · Sleeping bag · Space blanket · Change of rugged clothes · Flashlight & extra batteries · Pocket knife · Can opener · Heavy cord · Battery- or crank-operated weather and AM/FM radio · First aid kit · Sanitation kit · Medications & extra eyeglasses, hearing aid batteries, etc. · Whistle · Change of shoes & socks · Duct tape · Razor blades · Water filter · Water purification tablets · Solar charger · Battery pack · Crow bar · Utility shutoff tool · Fishing kit · Folding shovel · Reflective traffic vest · Lantern · Work gloves · Lighter or fire-starting kit

CAR GO BAG

Emergency rations (MREs, food bars, etc.) · Bottled water · Tent & tarp · Space blanket · Change of rugged clothes · Flashlight & extra batteries · Pocket knife · Can opener · Heavy cord · First-aid kit · Whistle · Change of shoes & socks · Duct tape · Razor blades · Water filter · Water purification tablets · Fishing kit · Folding shovel · Snow chains & a bag of sand · Jumper cables, flares, tow strap · Reflective traffic vest · Work gloves · Lighter or fire-starting kit

OFFICE GO BAG

Emergency rations (MREs, food bars, etc.) · Bottled water · Space blanket · Flashlight & extra batteries · Whistle · Change of shoes & socks · Reflective traffic vest

COMPACT EDC GO BAG

Flashlight & extra batteries · Pocket knife · Whistle · Phone charger battery pack · Lighter or fire-starting kit

124 KEEP IT IN YOUR POCKET

If you commute via public transit, are in school, or work in an environment where you don't have space to store a larger personal emergency kit, you may be limited to a pocket-based EDC kit. These highly compact kits are reasonably portable and designed to be carried on your person. If you assemble one yourself and it's so bulky that you don't like carrying it, revisit its contents and eliminate anything that's not absolutely necessary. The point of a pocket-based kit is to keep it in one; if it's not there, you won't have it handy should an emergency strike. On the other hand, if you consistently carry a purse, messenger bag, or backpack, you can add more items to your EDC kit—just don't make it so big that it becomes a nuisance to carry.

125 ASSEMBLE AN EDC

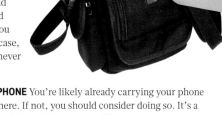

Everyday carry (EDC) refers to a small collection of tools, equipment, and supplies that are with you at all times to handle a variety of everyday and emergency situations. The list below represents a wide range of things you might carry. Tailor it to what's reasonable for your pockets, purse, briefcase, or school bag. Just remember, the more the better (within reason). You never know what item you might really need in a crisis.

TACTICAL FLASHLIGHT Useful for signaling and utility along with personal protection, a bright, durable, self defense-style flashlight is an essential part of your EDC gear.

MULTITOOL These come in several sizes, often with a knife. So, if you feel that carrying a separate knife is excessive, you still have a cutting tool.

POCKETKNIFE Even if you prefer not to carry a knife for self defense, there are a multitude of other reasons to have one, such as cooking, first aid, rescue, carving, and gear repair or adjustments.

WHISTLE Whistles can be used to call for help, warn anyone in earshot, and communicate with members of your group. Most are small and can be attached to a key ring.

BATTERY PACK Compact external batteries are small, usually a little longer than a tube of lipstick, and can carry enough power to give your phone a full charge. Add a short charging cable and you're set.

MARKER A permanent marker is an everyday object that you probably don't think about until you need one. These are water resistant and able to write on just about any surface. Find one with a clip that attaches easily to a key ring.

PARACORD Wristbands are one way to store and carry an emergency length of cord, but there are many others, such as a key chain fob or even shoelaces.

SMARTPHONE You're likely already carrying your phone everywhere. If not, you should consider doing so. It's a digital multitool that lets you call in emergencies, use apps, navigate, and access important files stored in the cloud.

SUNGLASSES Even when the weather is cloudy, consider carrying a decent pair of sunglasses with you. They can be worn as improvised safety glasses, and are useful when you need to rest but it's too bright to do so.

LIGHTER Even if you're not a smoker, a handy source of fire is useful in disaster situations when utilities are no longer functional, or for wilderness survival.

BANDANA This simple square of fabric can be employed as a tourniquet, a sling, a dust mask, and so much more.

STORAGE Consider placing your EDC kit into a small sturdy container for easy storage and organization. Also, include a compact stuff bag or folding pouch to add carrying capacity when it's needed; they can also be used for groceries and other everyday uses.

KEY RING STASH These small metal containers are perfect for storing extra emergency cash or a few doses of critical medication.

MINI FLASHLIGHT A tiny backup light is important in case your primary flashlight dies, or if you just need a little light. These utility lights can run for up to 15 hours.

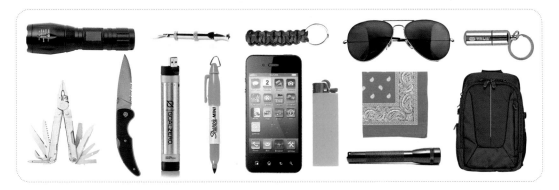

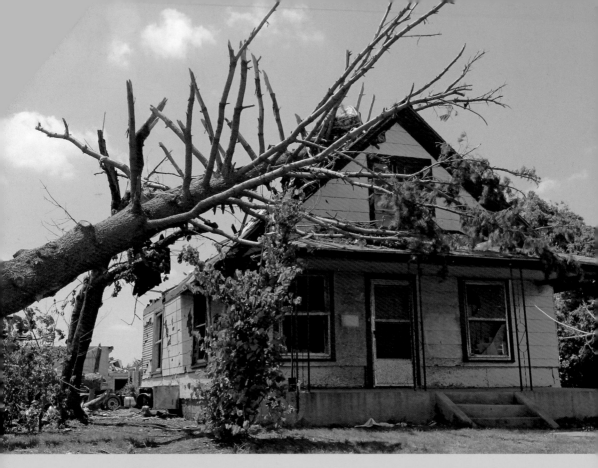

126 RIDE IT OUT AT HOME

If you're at home during an emergency or disaster, you're already one step ahead. After all, for those people at work or school, traveling or commuting, their number one concern is how to get home. You're already there. And that cliché about your home being your castle? In this event, it's your haven and your fortress, stocked with far more supplies than you'd have in your office or car kits. Of course, you'll also need to keep that castle safe and functional. Here is a checklist of important things to do after an emergency or disaster.

STEP 1 Examine your home. Is it damaged? How badly? Is it safe to be inside it? If you're not sure, then retreat outside and be prepared to set up camp in your yard until it's safe to go back in.

STEP 2 Shut off your utilities if you detect any damage, leaks, or smells.

STEP 3 Secure your pets.

STEP 4 Establish a reserve of water if your pipes still work. Fill your tub and as many water containers as you can in case the water gets cut off or rationed.

STEP 5 If you have lost power, set up your backup power supply or solar panels if they are in storage. If the power is still on, start charging all of your devices so that you'll be able to communicate if the power does go down.

STEP 6 Check if your landline phone and Internet access still work.

STEP 7 Turn on your radio or television to learn more about developments. Check the Internet for news and alerts for your area.

STEP 8 Contact family members and housemates to update them on the status of your home and family.

127 AVOID A RIOT

School campuses have become a regular focal point for protests, rallies, and, occasionally, riots. Regardless of whether any given protest is a peaceful political event, a disruptive strike, or an angry mob, it's smart to follow these guidelines to ensure your safety.

STEP 1 Stay indoors, away from windows and doorways.

STEP 2 Ask a teacher or staff member what to do, as there may already be an established school emergency action plan for such events.

STEP 3 Monitor social media such as Twitter and news apps for information about the protest.

STEP 4 Consider various exit routes from the building and different ways you can safely get home. Come up with at least three options.

STEP 5 If rioters start a fire nearby, or if the building you're in appears to be a focal point of the protest, it's time to leave. If possible, join up with a few people and calmly exit the building as a group, as far away from the center of the protest as possible.

STEP 6 Walk, don't run. Running attracts attention, and you might just be mistaken for a troublemaker by police. Hold hands or link elbows with your group to avoid getting separated. If you're caught up in the main body of the crowd, move with the crowd until you can escape onto a side street, or into a safe building.

STEP 7 Avoid public transportation routes that will move through or near the action, as you may end up getting trapped.

STEP 8 Do not approach police lines. You're unlikely to get through, and the risk for injury is greatest near the line between protesters and police.

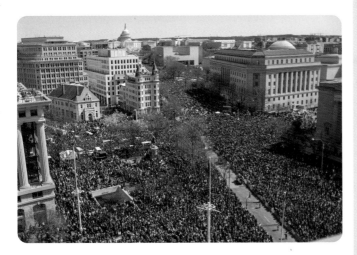

128 BE SCHOOL SAFE

One of the key considerations during an emergency at school is to memorize multiple exit routes, as well as several alternative ways to get home, should your usual route be unavailable. If it's not safe to leave the campus, knowing where safe shelter is can be equally important. Authorities should be able to assist, but you should know what to do if they can't.

A bag-based EDC is a natural choice for students. Note that schools often have strict weapons policies, so be sure to check your school's policies to avoid any problems if, say, your flashlight or pen knife are considered a threat.

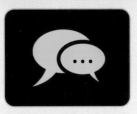

LIFE SAFETY APP
SOCIAL MEDIA

Social media is an easy way to communicate with your friends and family in the aftermath of a disaster or an accident. Plenty of people use social media every day, making it a logical go-to tool. Posting once is much faster and easier than texting or e-mailing everyone who might be concerned for your well-being. Even if you're not a current user, you should still consider signing up for one of these services to easily reach out when the time comes.

SUGGESTED APPS
• *Twitter*
• *Facebook*
• *Facebook Messenger*

129 ANTICIPATE EMERGENCIES AT WORK

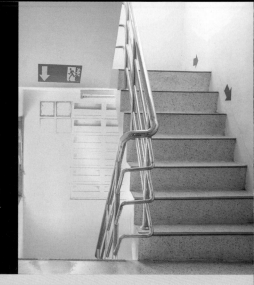

Many workplaces have some sort of emergency plan; the best prepared also take the time to rehearse them. Unfortunately, often a company has no process, or it's not well communicated. Once you know, you can either help to organize a plan, or at least know what you'll need to do personally to be prepared.

If you have your own office (or desk or other personal space), storing an emergency kit is easy. Otherwise, you'll likely be limited to just a pocket- or bag-based EDC kit. Based on how prepared your workplace is and what your own resources there will guide you as to what you can and should store as part of your office kit.

Next, you'll need to think about getting home. Plan out alternative routes and means for getting home *before* a disaster happens.

130 SURVIVE BEING STUCK IN AN ELEVATOR

Getting stuck in an elevator sounds scary, but typically the people in this situation are rescued within a few hours, so you'll likely be fine. Here are some steps to take if you are unlucky enough to feel the sudden lurch of an elevator stopping unexpectedly.

STEP 1 Use a cell phone or flashlight as a light source if the lights are out.

STEP 2 Try pressing each button on the panel; doing so may trigger normal operation again.

STEP 3 Try the emergency call button or use the emergency handset to call for assistance. Someone else in the building may also report the elevator as broken, and the elevator technician will be able to restore normal operation.

STEP 4 Check to see if your cellphone has service. If your signal is weak, try texting instead of calling; you're more likely to get a message through that way.

STEP 5 Try using a shoe to pound on the elevator door, or use a key or other metal object to create a sharp tapping sound if you're worried no one knows you're stuck.

STEP 6 Whether or not help is on the way, relax and get to know anyone sharing the elevator with you. If you keep gum, lozenges, or a food bar in your EDC kit, you can help stave off hunger if your rescue takes several hours.

STEP 7 Don't try to pry open the doors or attempt to escape through the ceiling hatch. Elevator doors have a fail-safe

locking mechanism, and in the elevator shaft you risk electrocution, falling, or being crushed. Wait to take any specific action unless you are prompted to do so by professional rescuers.

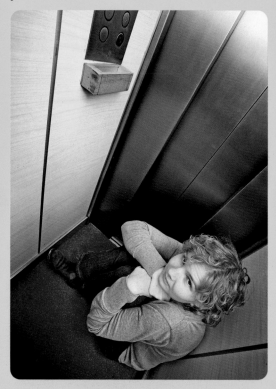

131 HAVE A COMMUTE BACKUP PLAN

If you're driving somewhere when a disaster strikes, one of your first actions should be to fill up your gas tank. After all, if the emergency goes on for some time, gas supplies may be limited or rationed. If the disaster occurs while you're on your way to work, you'll need to decide whether it makes more sense to return home or continue on to work. The best choice is probably to return home—you have more resources there and, of course, you'll want to be sure your home and family are safe.

Don't be foolish. If it's clear from listening to the radio or checking the Internet that returning home might put you in danger, head to the next safest place—which is likely your work. If you have a long or complex commute, pause for a moment to review your regular route and determine if there are any other safe places you could go to in the event of an emergency, such as another family member's home.

If you commute via public transit, and thus don't have a car emergency kit available, it might make sense to consider heading to your work to grab your office kit, if you think you might not be able to get home for a while.

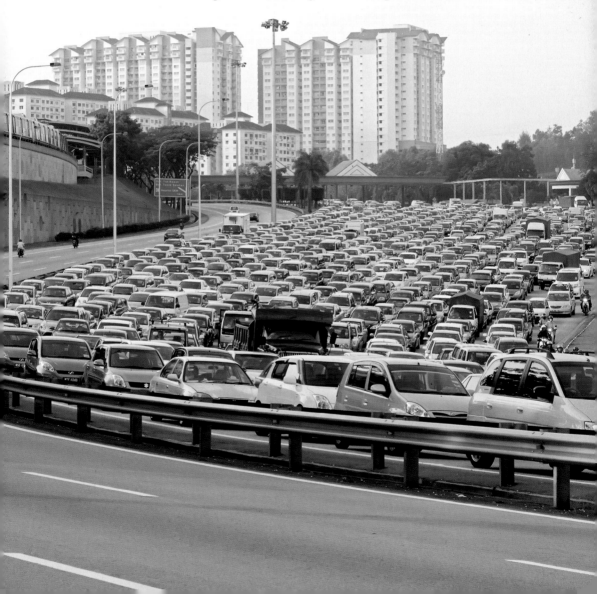

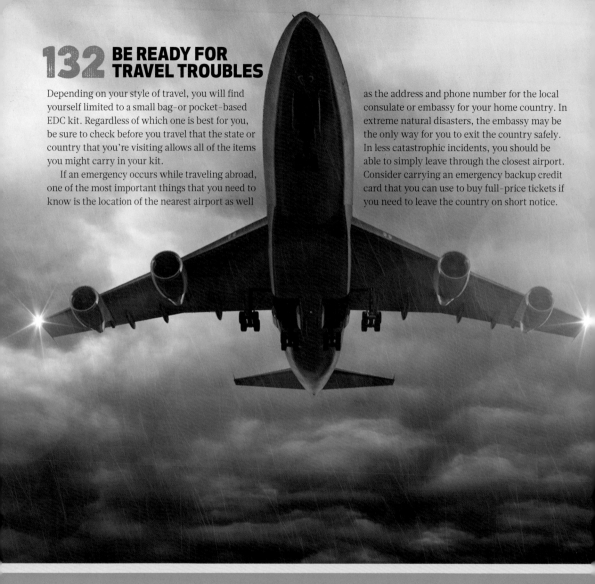

132 BE READY FOR TRAVEL TROUBLES

Depending on your style of travel, you will find yourself limited to a small bag- or pocket-based EDC kit. Regardless of which one is best for you, be sure to check before you travel that the state or country that you're visiting allows all of the items you might carry in your kit.

If an emergency occurs while traveling abroad, one of the most important things that you need to know is the location of the nearest airport as well as the address and phone number for the local consulate or embassy for your home country. In extreme natural disasters, the embassy may be the only way for you to exit the country safely. In less catastrophic incidents, you should be able to simply leave through the closest airport. Consider carrying an emergency backup credit card that you can use to buy full-price tickets if you need to leave the country on short notice.

133 GET A NEW PASSPORT

If you're traveling for a long time or going through a high-risk area, an emergency replacement passport kit can save a lot of frustration. Your kit should have a paper photocopy of your passport and visas, along with two passport photos and a printed copy of your itinerary. Include an alternative photo ID, such as a driver's license, and proof of citizenship, such as a copy of your birth certificate or certificate of naturalization. If your passport is stolen, you may need to file a police report prior to applying for a replacement passport. Upload pictures of your passport and visas into a cloud storage service—along with a police report if at all possible—so you can retrieve your files from any computer or smartphone. Finally, be sure to store the kit separately from your passport; you don't want to lose it, too!

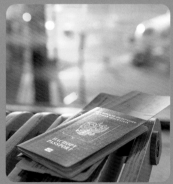

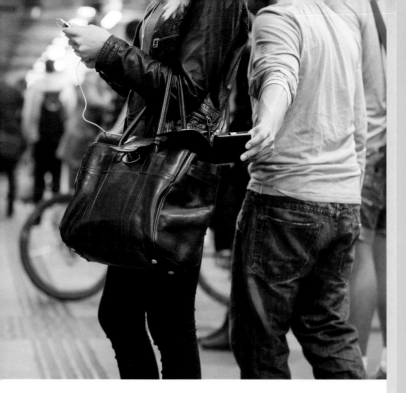

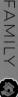

135
AVOID BEING A VICTIM

Don't just check for where your valuables are with a pat; put your hand in your pocket with your wallet and keep it there. If you're carrying a purse, sling it over your shoulder and tightly clamp down on it with your arm. Sling bags that keep your belongings toward your front are great.

While you're traveling, carry belongings in bags and wallets that have slash-resistant mesh, and use cables or chains to attach to fixed objects or your person. Store your passport, credit cards, and the majority of your money inside a hidden pouch such as a money belt. Don't carry bags on your back or wallets in your back pocket. If you carry a bag with many zippers, use small locks or screw-gate carabiners to make the bag harder to open.

134 SPOT A PICKPOCKET

Whether traveling abroad or commuting via public transit, you are pretty much always at some risk of being pick pocketed. High-risk areas can include major tourism sites, museums, restaurants, cafés, bars, parks, and the beach. The risk increases abroad; as a tourist, professional pickpockets see you as an easy mark, since you're more likely to be carrying valuables such as cash or credit cards.

The first step to successful pickpocketing is finding a reason to get very close to you; if you suddenly feel like someone is uncomfortably close, raise your guard and get out of there. Engaging them creates an opportunity for them to victimize you. Trust your instincts and use your situational awareness to avoid this situation as much as possible. Common pickpocket tactics include the following.

- "Accidentally" bumping into you or jostling you on the street
- Standing too close to you on public transit or crowding up against you while both of you are passing through a turnstile
- Asking for directions while holding a large map close to you (to hide an accomplice from your field of view)
- Asking for the time, or for a light for a cigarette
- Trying to sell you something
- Spilling something on you and then offering to clean it off
- Dropping groceries, coins, or other items in front of you
- A crowd of young children suddenly surrounding you and demanding your attention
- An overly friendly and attractive woman who appears to be drunk
- An overly helpful stranger offering to take you where you need to go

136
USE A DECOY WALLET

To foil pickpockets, carry a decoy wallet or purse with a little bit of money and a few random items inside so it seems legit. Put it inside an obvious pocket or carry it conspicuously so that it will be taken rather than your real wallet or purse. Don't put in any fake money or anything that will obviously tip off the thief that their prize was a decoy, or they may come back in anger to find your real valuables, to hurt you, or both.

137 PACK LIFEBOAT RATIONS

If you're stranded in your car somewhere you can't call or walk out, your car effectively becomes a lifeboat until help arrives. This is where your car disaster kit plays a major role in keeping you alive until help arrives. Two items key to your survival will be your food stash and your water supply. However, your car is likely to experience temperature extremes, especially since your trunk (the likely storage space) isn't climate controlled. Extremes of temperature can significantly reduce shelf life.

You need to create a kit that can be stored for years in your car without having to worry that your food or water has gone bad. Lifeboat rations are a good, rarely-thought-of option. These are designed for storage in harsh conditions and have a shelf life of about five years. While you may want to also keep other food and water to supplement the rations, having these as the minimum ensures you have enough food and water to hold out for a few days.

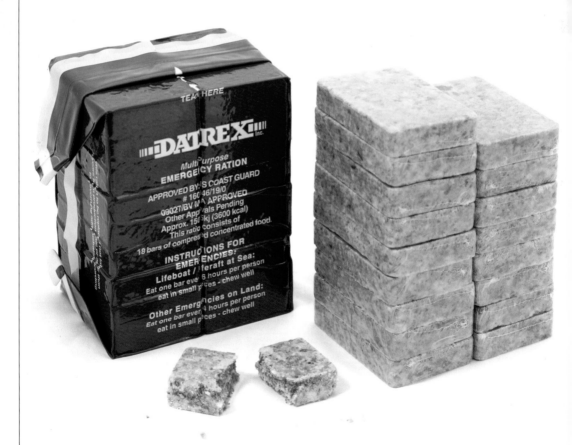

138 GET THE RIGHT RATIONS

There are some general considerations to keep in mind when you're shopping for that easy-to-store food stash. You'll want your rations to be compact in size for easy storage, and have a long shelf life (about five years is typical). They also have to be durable and in sturdy packaging such as sealed heavy plastic or foil containers.

The rations should be divided into easy-to-grasp portions. For food, rations are usually kept in 3,600-calorie packages, subdivided into portions of 200 to 400 calories. Water usually comes in individual ration pouches of about 4 ounces each.

Rations also should be designed for conditions where the water supply is limited. This means water should be included for drinking, and the foodstuffs should all be ready to eat, not requiring any preparation or cooking.

139 ADD PROTEIN

Lifeboat rations are designed to keep you alive in conditions where you have a limited water supply and don't need to exert yourself. This is perfect if you're stranded with your car but isn't as useful if your goal is to hike out. So if you're fit, inclined to leave your car to find help, and have a backpack-based kit in your car for easy carrying, be sure to add more proteins to your car kit in the form of jerky, canned fish, or protein bars. The downside, of course, is that the shelf life of such items is much more limited and will require regular inspections to make sure the food is still safe.

140 SIGNAL FOR HELP

No matter how you decide to try and attract attention, when it comes to signaling, your best bet is to get to out the largest clearing at the highest elevation that you can easily reach. If you're stranded with your vehicle and using it as a lifeboat, then you'll want to find a location that's reasonably close so that search parties can match your signal with your location. There are a few different ways to do this.

BUILD A FIRE It's likely that the easiest and most commonly thought of way to signal is with fire. You can build your own signal fire in a large clearing ahead of time, and then wait until you are certain someone is within sight of the smoke, which is the most visible part of the fire. Light a hot blaze, and then cover it up with plenty of greenery. If there's a lone dead tree standing in that clearing, sacrifice it to create a torch visible for miles.

LIGHT A FLARE Pen flares—part of a pilot's survival vest— will fire a small signal flare several hundred feet into the air. Larger flares or flare guns can achieve even greater heights with a more visible signal. You should treat these as essential emergency supplies, but be very careful in dry areas, as you might inadvertently ignite a grass or forest fire that may well further endanger you.

USE A MIRROR Reflective materials are some of the easiest survival tools to carry and use. If you have a mirror designed specifically for signaling to aircraft, follow the directions printed on its back. For a regular mirror, or other reflective material, hold it at an angle that allows you to see the light reflected on the ground, then slowly bring it up to eye level and aim at your target. For best results, try tilting or rotating it slightly, which will flash to a search party.

GO HIGH TECH Radio and GPS technology can mean the difference between life and death when stranded. Consider investing in a GPS signaling device that can transmit your location as well as send text messages. These aren't cheap, and frequently require a subscription, but they can really pay off. A satellite phone or two-way radio can also call for help on emergency frequencies; it also has the added benefit of being useful for camping and other outdoor activities.

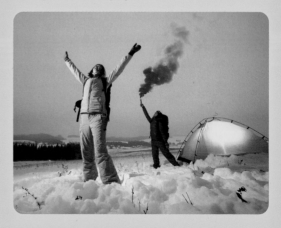

141 IDENTIFY DISASTER RISKS AND NEEDS

Before you can write a plan you need to know what you're planning for. These guidelines give you a good foundation for your emergency preparedness.

STEP 1 Identify the various types of natural disasters that are possible in your area as well as potential man-made risks. For example, are you near a freeway, rail line, port, factory, or industrial facility? These can all be a source of hazardous materials incidents. Consider how you might have to prepare for each type of disaster that might happen.

STEP 2 Learn about the available public warning systems in your area. Are sirens used? If so, learn what the different signals mean during an emergency. Some cities or counties require signing up for any text, e-mail, or smartphone app notifications of disasters, while others will automatically call your landline phone.

STEP 3 Do you have pets? If so, learn what local resources are available to help you out in an emergency. For example, many shelters don't allow pets, so you may have to create a separate plan for caring for your animals.

STEP 4 If you have children, ask school administrators about their disaster plans so you know what you can expect. For elderly or disabled people, check with their health care providers for assistance in planning.

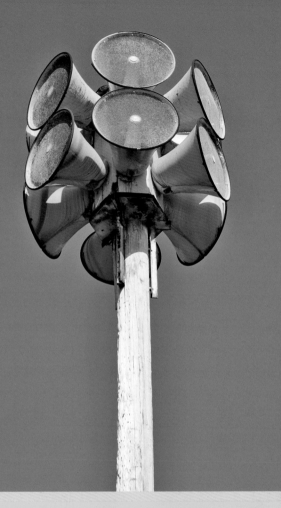

142 PREPARE FOR A ZOMBIE ATTACK

You might have seen news stories a few years ago about how the United States government was preparing for the zombie apocalypse. Much as that sounds like a typical crazy conspiracy theory (or the plot of a late-night movie), in this case it's actually true . . . sort of.

What actually happened is that the U.S. Centers for Disease Control and Prevention, one of America's prime sources for helpful disaster preparedness information and resources, came up with a website, a comic book, and a full publicity campaign to get kids (and zombie-loving hipsters) excited about understanding emergency preparedness.

Since it's important to involve everyone in yours household in the disaster-planning process in order for your efforts to be successful, why not try engaging teens and tweens (and zombie-loving adults) by using these free downloadable materials? The materials cover such essentials as putting together a first-aid kit, ensuring sanitary conditions, stocking up on safe food and water—all the stuff we're discussing in this book, except with the added bonus of the undead. And if the zombies do rise up? Bonus, you're that much more prepared!

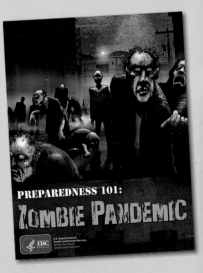

PREPAREDNESS 101:
ZOMBIE PANDEMIC

CDC U.S. Department of Health and Human Services
Centers for Disease Control and Prevention

143 DEVELOP A PLAN

Once you've assessed the likelihood of various disasters in your area and taken a good look at your household's needs, you're ready to start developing a detailed disaster plan.

First, meet with your household and discuss the need to prepare for disaster. If you have younger children, you'll want to explain dangers to them in an age-appropriate way. Plan how the group can best share responsibilities and work together as a team.

Be sure your plan is succinct. Create an outline, not a novel, with just enough detail to be practical. Plans with too much detail can be burdensome during a disaster. Discuss the types of disasters that are most likely to happen, local warning systems, and any expected challenges with infants, pets, and elderly or disabled members of your household. Explore what to do in each situation. Everyone should know and have access to the plan. Consider e-mailing a copy to all members of the household or using cloud storage for easy access on any computer or device.

Determine at least two home escape routes, and agree upon a meeting point away from the home in case of a local emergency, like a fire. Consider some evacuation routes outside the area in case of a more significant incident.

In case family members are separated at the time of an incident, include a section of the plan for how to reunite. Separation is a real possibility when adults are at work and children are at school.

Develop an emergency communication plan. Ask an out-of-town relative or friend to be your family contact who can coordinate communication in case other means fail. If unable to reach one another, family members should call the contact and tell them where they are and how they are doing. Include the contact's name, address, e-mail, and phone number in your plan.

144 CHECK OUT YOUR PLAN

Part of the planning process includes a few universal steps that all households can take, including the items on this checklist.

☐ Post a list of direct-dial emergency telephone numbers (ambulance, fire, police, and so on) by landline phones and load them into the address book of your mobile phones.

☐ Make sure that everyone in your household knows how to turn off the various utility mains—electricity, gas, and water.

☐ Thoroughly check your home for any potential hazards.

☐ Do an inventory of your pantry. Stock emergency food and water.

☐ Assemble a disaster kit for your home and go bags for all members of the household.

☐ Consider establishing safe rooms for disasters that might affect your home

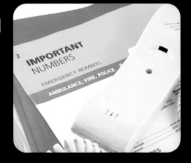

☐ Make some copies of all important documents, such as birth and marriage certificates, deeds, titles, wills, and trusts. Keep one copy in a home fire safe and put another copy in a safety deposit box or with a trusted relative who lives outside the area. Consider scanning the files and storing them in the cloud or on a flash drive.

☐ Evaluate your insurance to see what disaster types are covered or excluded. Get coverage for those you reasonably anticipate in your area. Document all valuables, including serial number, make, and model in case you need to file a claim after a disaster. Consider adding copies of any related original receipts to your archive.

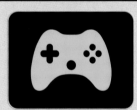

145 KEEP IN CONTACT

It's important that everyone in your household knows the plan for getting in touch with everyone else after a disaster. Even if you've loaded all the information into your mobile phones, consider also keeping a paper copy in case your phone is dead when you need the information.

Include the contact information for each member of your household; make sure that it lists their full name, relation to the family, work and/or school address and phone number, mobile phone number, their e-mail address, and any other contact info that might be relevant.

Don't forget to include important information, such as date of birth, medical insurance policy, blood type, allergies, or medical conditions. Also add names and contact information for any designated out-of-town family contacts.

List muster or evacuation points from your family plan. Review and update the information in the plan annually. Additionally, ensure all members of your household have ICE entries (see item 147).

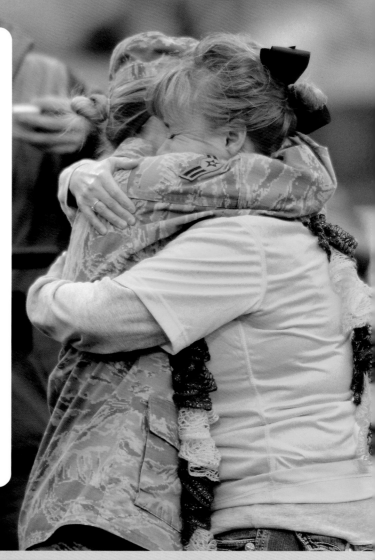

146 COMMUNICATE IN A DISASTER

During a regional emergency or disaster, mobile phone systems quickly become overloaded with voice calls. If you cannot get through, try text messaging instead, as that has a much higher chance of getting through during those circumstances.

If you want to communicate to everyone easily with a single step, consider posting to Twitter, Facebook, or other social media with your status. Alternatively, the Red Cross offers a free "Safe and Well" online listing service. Just be sure to plan with other members of your household which of these systems you'll use should you not be reachable by phone.

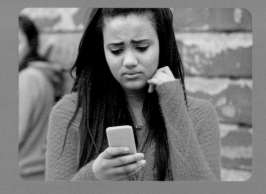

147 BE AWARE OF ICE

"In case of emergency," or ICE, is a concept that came about in 2005 when it became apparent that mobile phones were ubiquitous and were a great way to inform doctors and emergency responders whom to contact in a crisis, simply by programming extra address book entries into their cell phone, such as "ICE, dad" or "ICE, wife."

These days, assuming that you are carrying a smartphone, it's a little more complicated since your screen is probably locked. However, both Android and iOS phones are able to show a list of designated emergency contacts from the lock screen.

Other options include putting a sticker on the back of your phone or ID with a list of your ICE contacts, or printing out an ICE card that you can put in your wallet, purse, or glove compartment (see item 148, below).

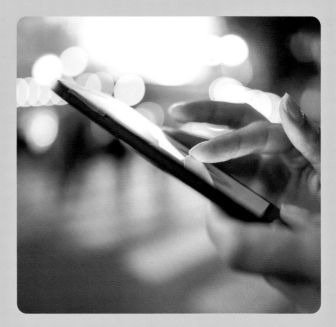

148 CARRY A CARD

Many insurance companies and automobile associations offer free versions of an ICE card that you can download and carry in your wallet or glove box. Or you can photocopy or scan and fill out the one provided here, to make things easier for first responders, and for you and your loved ones in case of an emergency.

ICE IN CASE OF EMERGENCY — OUTDOOR LIFE

VEHICLE DRIVERS

PRIMARY (FULL NAME): _____

SECONDARY (FULL NAME): _____

ICE CONTACTS

PHYSICIAN: _____ ALLERGY(S): _____

MEDICAL CONDITION(S): _____

NAME/RELATION: _____

PHONE 1: _____ PHONE 2: _____

NAME/RELATION: _____

PHONE 1: _____ PHONE 2: _____

NAME/RELATION: _____

PHONE 1: _____ PHONE 2: _____

ICE IN CASE OF EMERGENCY

NAME: _____

ICE CONTACTS

PHYSICIAN: _____

ALLERGY(S): _____

MEDICAL CONDITION(S): _____

NAME/RELATION: _____

PHONE 1: _____

PHONE 2: _____

NAME/RELATION: _____

PHONE 1: _____

PHONE 2: _____

NAME/RELATION: _____

PHONE 1: _____

PHONE 2: _____

149 MITIGATE HOME DISASTER

Use this easy reference guide to check off the various things you can do to reduce the risk or severity of the problems you're likely to encounter in the event of the most common natural disasters.

DISASTER

- BASIC SAFETY
- EARTHQUAKE
- FLOODING
- HIGH WINDS
- FIRE
- FREEZING

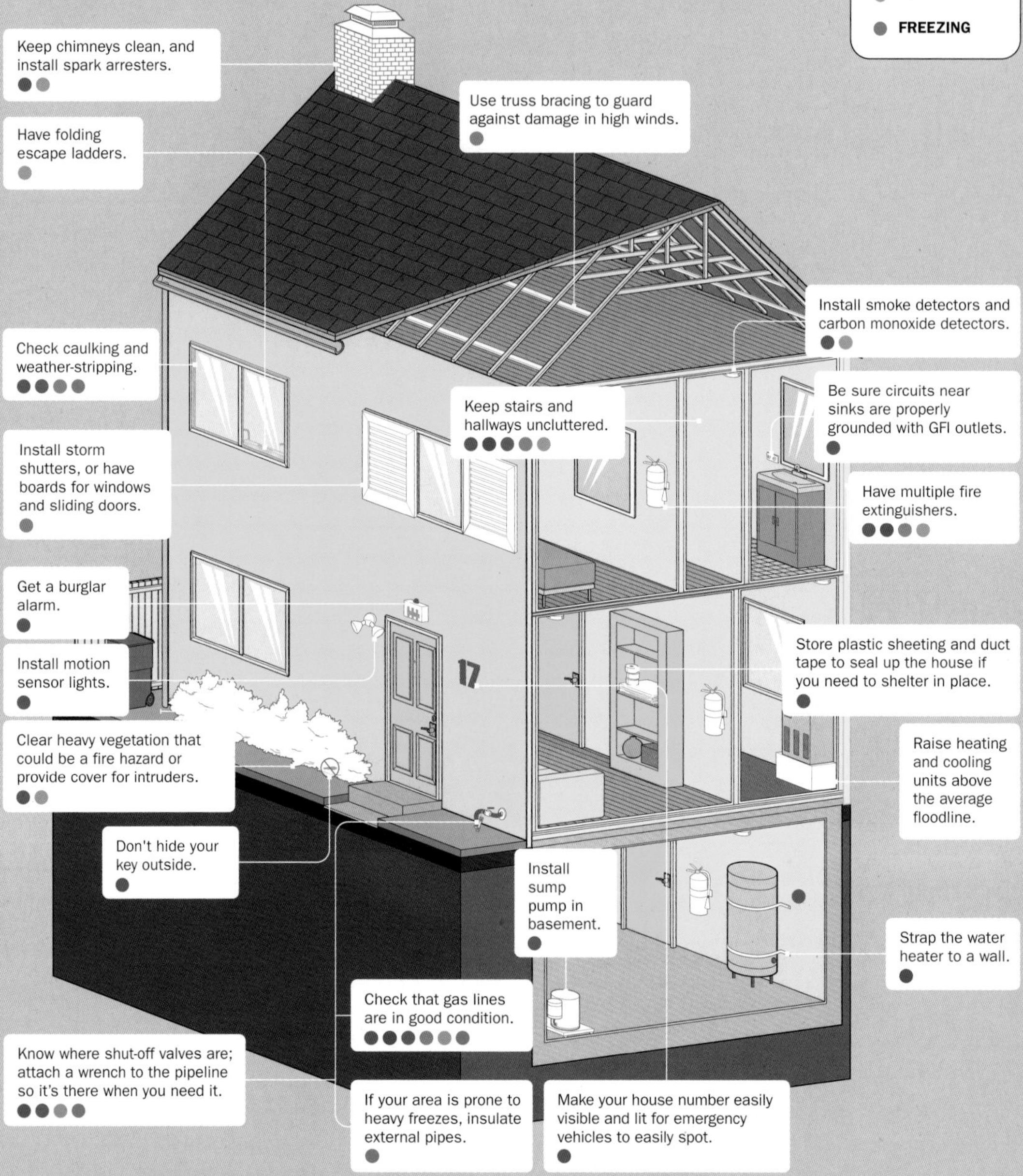

Keep chimneys clean, and install spark arresters.

Have folding escape ladders.

Use truss bracing to guard against damage in high winds.

Install smoke detectors and carbon monoxide detectors.

Check caulking and weather-stripping.

Keep stairs and hallways uncluttered.

Be sure circuits near sinks are properly grounded with GFI outlets.

Install storm shutters, or have boards for windows and sliding doors.

Have multiple fire extinguishers.

Get a burglar alarm.

Store plastic sheeting and duct tape to seal up the house if you need to shelter in place.

Install motion sensor lights.

Clear heavy vegetation that could be a fire hazard or provide cover for intruders.

Raise heating and cooling units above the average floodline.

Don't hide your key outside.

Install sump pump in basement.

Strap the water heater to a wall.

Know where shut-off valves are; attach a wrench to the pipeline so it's there when you need it.

Check that gas lines are in good condition.

If your area is prone to heavy freezes, insulate external pipes.

Make your house number easily visible and lit for emergency vehicles to easily spot.

17

150 KEEP IT TOGETHER

If you keep your camping gear down in the basement, your disaster supplies in a closet, and your tools in your garage, you're not unusual—but you're also at a disadvantage in an emergency. Instead, store your tools and camping gear with your disaster supplies. You can easily grab items as you need them for, say, a camping trip or DIY project, but you won't have to scramble for essentials in an emergency, especially difficult if your home is partially destroyed or inaccessible. Consider buying some large sturdy plastic storage tubs, keep everything labeled and organized, and don't forget to return anything you "borrow" from your stash. If you should need to evacuate quickly, you can just grab the tubs and go.

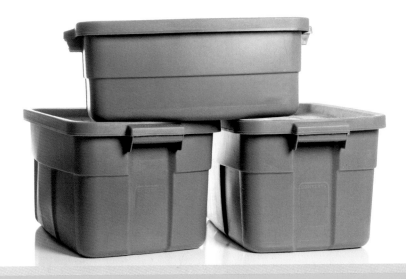

151 FUEL UP

In any emergency, you'll want to be sure your car is gassed up and ready to go. Get in the habit of filling your tank as soon as it drops below half a tank, especially if you're anticipating storms or other severe weather that might knock out power to the area. Without electricity, gas pumps won't work, and once the power comes back on, there's likely to be a run on the stations as everyone rushes to refuel.

For additional security, or if you fear that power might be down for a significant period, you might want to store extra fuel at home (for your cars, a generator, or maybe a chain saw). If you choose to do this, it's important to store the fuel safely, as not only is it highly flammable, but the fumes can be dangerous. Always store gas in approved airtight containers that do not vent, and store all those containers in a grounded double-walled steel flammable safety cabinet.

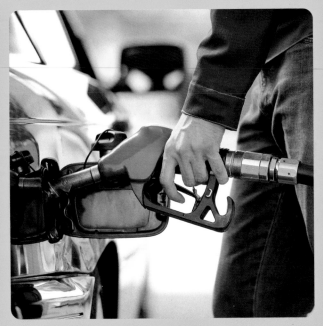

152 KEEP A WEEK'S SUPPLY

In a serious disaster, local emergency resources will be overloaded. Supplies from regional disaster caches, the Red Cross, and other agencies will take at least 72 hours, but expect longer delays, to arrive in the affected area. So, when planning a disaster kit, consider five to seven days' supplies the minimum to have on hand. If you live in a disaster-prone area, such as flood plains, tornado alley, or near an earthquake fault, consider keeping enough supplies for a week or more, depending on your ability to easily store and manage a larger cache.

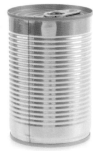

153 STOCK THE RIGHT SUPPLIES

A dedicated food cache will ensure you have enough to survive longer term. Include a variety of foods, including those that do not require cooking, water, or special preparation. Incorporate some comfort foods and treats that have a long shelf life, such as hard candy, to add variety. Ensure that you've accounted for anyone in your household with dietary restrictions.

Store everything in a cool, dry place. Keep boxed foods in airtight plastic or metal containers to protect it from pests and to extend its shelf life. Write the date each item was placed into storage on its packaging to easily determine how long it's been stored. At a minimum, review all supplies annually. Consider reviewing your food supplies every six months, when you're rotating your water supply. Throw out any canned goods that become swollen, dented, rusted, or corroded.

154 CONSIDER EMERGENCY ALTERNATIVES

Emergency supplies should be nonperishable and able to keep for years. Here are the most common options to consider.

FOOD SOURCE	ADVANTAGE	DISADVANTAGE	NOTES
FREEZE DRIED	Very long shelf life	Require water to prepare	Generally considered the best option for taste
CANNED	Inexpensive	Bulky	Problematic in freezing conditions or high humidity (danger of rust)
MRE	Packaged for convenience	Expensive	Taste can be monotonous
DRY GOODS (wheat, rice, corn, sugar, pinto beans, oats, pasta, potato flakes, nonfat powdered milk)	Very long shelf life	Require preparation for storage and usually need other ingredients to cook	Not generally appropriate for shorter-term emergencies
FOOD BARS/JERKY	Portable, easy to eat	Shorter shelf life	Not a satisfying substitute for a meal

155 HOLD YOUR WATER

Depending on the situation, tap water may not be available or may not be safe to drink. Therefore you need to have a back-up supply. There are three basic ways to store your water, each with its own advantages and disadvantages. The best disaster kits will rely on a combination of these various resources; regardless of which type of containers you use, always store your water in a cool, dark place. You may also end up needing to rely on secondary sources of water, such as your water heater or collecting rainwater.

WATER SOURCE	ADVANTAGE	DISADVANTAGE
EMERGENCY WATER RATIONS	Long shelf life	Expensive
STORE-BOUGHT WATER JUGS	Easy to manage	Short shelf life
REUSABLE FOOD-GRADE WATER JUGS	Uses tap water	Container must be cleaned and sterilized

156 KEEP CAFFEINE ON HAND

Caffeine can be a vital supplement to your disaster kit, particularly when access to water, a stove, and the time to prepare coffee or tea are not an option. Luckily there are alternatives for a pick-me-up: caffeinated gum and caffeine pills. Neither requires preparation, and they're both compact and easily carried in your go bag, but gum has the added advantage of helping suppress hunger a bit, which may be useful if you're trying to conserve food supplies.

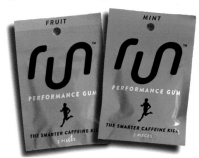

157 TEST YOUR KIT

The only way to know for sure if all your supplies will actually last five to seven days is to do a test. This is best done on a long weekend right before rotating supplies that will expire shortly. It's important that everyone in the household understands the need to avoid cheating by buying outside food or eating out, as that can lead to a false idea of how long your supplies will last. Another reason to test out your kit of emergency supplies? Children who are stressed or traumatized after a disaster may refuse to eat strange foods; this provides a chance to taste-test things first.

STEP 1 Gather your household and discuss the test, so that everyone can be involved.

STEP 2 Secretly pick a date several months away for the test to happen.

STEP 3 On that date, declare an "emergency", and that whatever food and water is in the house is all you have to live on for the next five to seven days.

STEP 4 See how long your household can last on your disaster supplies and the available food in your fridge, freezer, and pantry.

STEP 5 Restock disaster supplies and perishable foods.

STEP 6 Enjoy a nice meal out to celebrate.

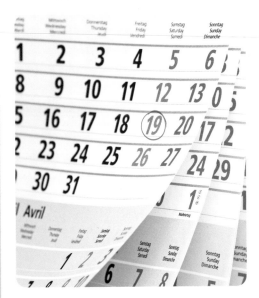

158 STOCK FOOD AND WATER

Even if you're really well prepared, you may end up utilizing tips from the improvised set of suggestions as a way of extending your water and food supply in the event of a longer-lasting disaster.

WATER
- Emergency water rations in disaster supplies (5-year shelf life).

- 7-gallon (26.5 liter) potable water jugs (rotated every 6 months and sanitized between uses)

- Filled reusable water bottles in go bags (rotated every 6 months and sanitized between uses)

- Extra cases of coconut water or sports drinks (rotated every year or per expiration date)

FOOD
- Military style MREs in disaster supplies (3- to 5-year shelf life)

- Freeze-dried (20- to 25-year shelf life) and canned goods (1- to 2-year shelf life) stored securely

- Food bars and dried meats (rotated annually or according to expiration date)

- Emergency rations in go bags (rotated annually)

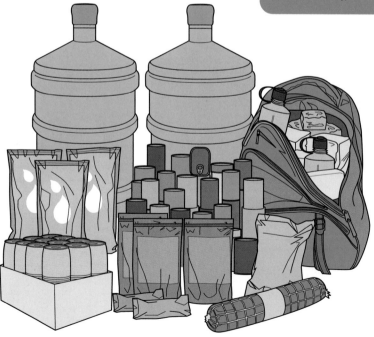

If you haven't been able to put together a proper set of food and water supplies for a disaster, or are in a situation where you can't get to the stocks you have, you can still improvise. Here are some suggestions.

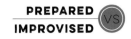
IMPROVISED

FOOD
- Whatever food you have in your fridge and pantry, carefully rationed until help arrives
- Whatever food is available for purchase at stores that might still be open
- Whatever fruits and vegetables might be ripe in your garden

WATER
- Melted ice from freezers
- From the water heater
- From filling bathtub after the disaster (if there is any water pressure available)
- From rain or snow (to purify see item 241)

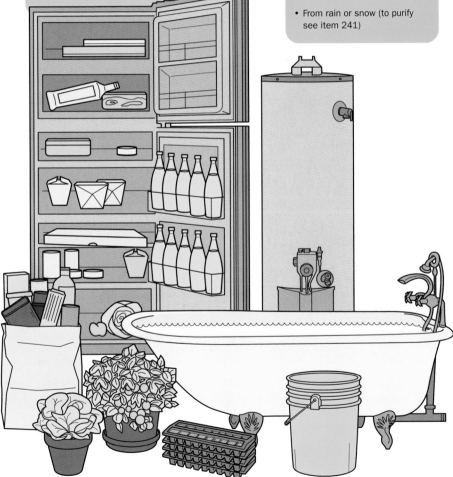

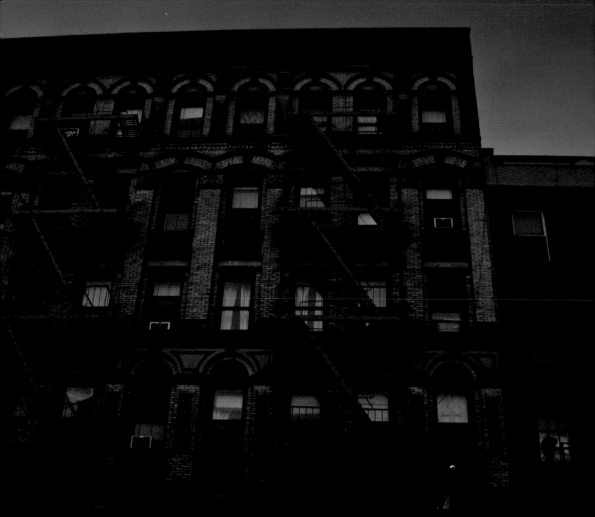

159 GET READY FOR LIGHTS OUT

Blackouts are common in both summer and winter. In some areas of the country, the middle to end of summer is known as "blackout season," as climate-control demands on the power supply tend to overload providers. In the peak of the winter season, ice and storms can bring down power lines. And year-round, blackouts can also be caused by lightning strikes, solar flares, substation failures, or fires. No matter what the cause, there are things you can do when this inevitably happens in your hood.

First, turn off anything that was on when the blackout began, to avoid taxing the electrical grid when power comes back. Leave one light or radio on so you'll know right away when the power is restored. Use an uninterruptible power supply (UPS) for any computers or critical electronics; this will power your devices even when the power is off and protect against power surges. Use surge protectors (not to be confused with a simple power strip) to protect any electronics not connected to a UPS.

If you use cordless phones for your landline, purchase a regular corded model that doesn't require power. These usually keep working after the power goes out and are still the best way to reach emergency services. Keep some cash available, either in a small safe or hidden away in a lockbox; ATMs and cash registers won't work during a blackout.

Stock up on batteries and, if you live in a blackout-prone area, you should consider investing in a solar- or gas-powered generator. Secure any generator with a cable lock or chain, as it may be a target for theft by the less prepared and larcenous. Have fun while you wait with board games, puzzles, charades, cards, and crafts.

160 GUARD THE NEIGHBORHOOD

When your entire neighborhood is dark, those familiar streets may suddenly seem ominous. But there is strength in numbers, especially if you've made the effort of getting to know your neighbors. If you're new to your neighborhood or haven't yet met your neighbors, you can use disaster preparedness as the perfect excuse to do so. Here are some things that your neighborhood can coordinate together.

PHONE IT IN Create a neighborhood phone list with both landlines and mobile numbers. Circulate it via e-mail so everyone has each others' e-mail as well.

HAM IT UP See if anyone in your neighborhood is a HAM operator, and agree in advance what frequencies to use to communicate. Alternatively, everyone in the neighborhood can coordinate on the cheap and nearly ubiquitous Family Radio Service (FRS) radios that don't require a license to operate.

SET A WATCH Create a neighborhood watch program if one doesn't already exist for your immediate area. If one does, join it and also advocate to create a blackout plan for the neighborhood.

CHECK IN As part of your neighborhood disaster plan, you can add a standard practice of neighbors checking in on each other to make sure everything is okay. If your neighbor is not home at the time, you can also be a good neighbor by keeping an eye on their property for them.

GO ON PATROL In a blackout, have a neighborhood watch group patrol the area to keep an eye on things and to deter opportunistic criminals.

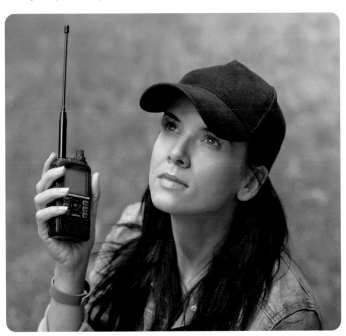

161 EAT RIGHT IN AN OUTAGE

Food can spoil quickly during an extended power outage, and having a plan for how to consume your perishables will help prevent any foodborne illness. Here's how to prioritize what to consume first.

First, use perishable foods from the refrigerator before they spoil. An unopened fridge will keep foods cold for about 4 hours, so keep the doors closed as much as possible.

Next, consume food from the freezer. A full freezer will stay cold for about 48 hours (24 hours if it is half full) if the door remains closed.

If it looks like the power outage will continue beyond a day, prepare a camping cooler with ice for your freezer items.

Use canned items, dry goods, and nonperishable foods last, as they will stay edible the longest.

162 THROW IT OUT IF IT'S THAWED

Throw away any food that has been exposed to temperatures above 40°F (4°C) for 2 hours or longer, or that has an unusual odor, color, or texture. Don't rely on taste or appearance to determine whether it's safe for you to eat.

If the food in the freezer is colder than 40°F (4°C) and has ice crystals, you can refreeze it. If you are not sure whether food is cold enough, take its temperature by using a food thermometer. When in doubt, throw it out!

163

COMMUNICATE CLEARLY

In an extended power outage or other disaster, it's likely that your landline, cell phone, or Internet connection will stop working. Here are some items you can use to keep you safe and communicating with others.

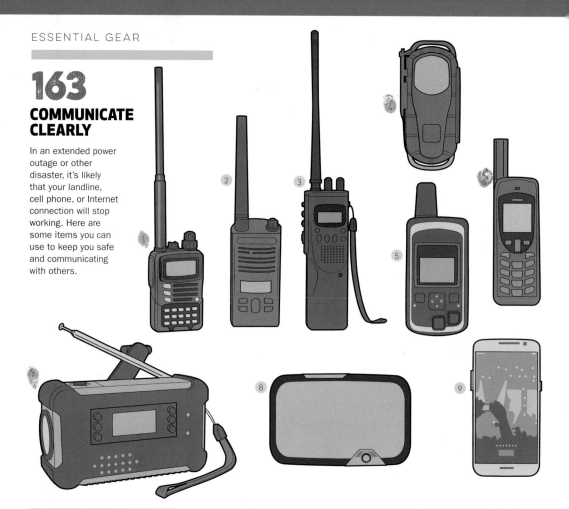

HAM RADIO Amateur radio might seem almost quaint, but during a disaster, HAM radio is often one of the most reliable ways to communicate with others and call for help. Handheld radios have a limited range, however, a network of free repeaters can extend coverage over hundreds of miles, and base stations with large antennas can communicate globally, but you'll need to get a license.

MURS RADIO Multi-Use Radio Service (MURS) is the big brother to the inexpensive Family Radio Service (FRS) devices in common use today on ski slopes and camping trips. Both types are license-free, but MURS has better range and is less crowded with other users. Neither radio type has a formal emergency channel; however, they can provide easy and inexpensive communication for neighborhood watch and other groups.

CITIZEN'S BAND RADIO CB radios have a highly dedicated following even though the older technology suffers from poorer audio quality than its modern cousins, the handheld range is relatively small, and the units tend to be bulky. However, CB channel 9 is a monitored emergency channel that can be used to call for help, which makes CB still relevant in areas with no cell coverage.

PERSONAL LOCATOR BEACONS PLBs have their origins in maritime and aviation search and rescue. Once modern electronics decreased the size of a unit to that of a large cell phone, it was possible for portable applications like hiking or backcountry skiing to make use of the technology. By combining a radio transmitter and GPS receiver, a PLB first sends a unique code that identifies you and then broadcasts a homing signal to allow planes to find your location. You may be billed for the cost of your rescue.

SATELLITE MESSENGERS Using the same technology and network

DEVICE	TYPICAL COST	MONTHLY FEES	LICENCE REQUIRED	DEPENDABLE AVERAGE RANGE (MILES)	POWER (WATTS)	VOICE/TEXT
HAM (UHF)	$200–300	None	Yes	3[1]	5	Yes/No/Yes[2]
MURS	$100–200	None	No	2	2	Yes/No/No
GMRS	$50	None	Yes	1	5	Yes/No/No
FRS	$25	None	No	<1	0.5	Yes/No/No
CB	$100	None	No	2	5	Yes/No/No
PLB	$150–300	None	No	Global	N/A	No/No/No
SATELLITE PHONE	$200–1000	Yes	No	Global	N/A	Yes/Yes/Yes
SATELLITE MESSENGER	$200–300	Yes	No	Global	N/A	No/Yes/Yes
BLUETOOTH MESSAGING	Free	None	No	200 feet	N/A	No/Yes/Yes

[1] Can be extended to hundreds of miles/km with repeaters.　[2] Requires additional hardware.

as satellite phones, these compact devices are used similarly to a PLB to call for help, send text messages, and transmit their location so others can track the user on a website. They are popular with hikers and long-distance travelers who don't need the function or expense of a full satellite phone.

6 SATELLITE PHONE The per-minute cost of a satellite call is much higher than that of a regular cell phone—but worth it in an emergency. Intended for areas where there is no cell phone coverage, they're also extremely helpful when a disaster affects the local phone infrastructure. If you need one temporarily, plenty of companies rent them for short-term use.

7 HAND-CRANKED RADIO No longer just a type of AM/FM/weather radio, these handy devices are also a functional hub with multiple charging options (including AC, DC, battery, solar, and USB), a flashlight, a USB port for charging small electronics, audio jacks for use as an external speaker, and a versatile part of every home disaster kit.

8 WIRELESS HOTSPOTS These are useful in everyday settings, but when your internet connection is lost due to infrastructure damage, it can take a long time online. If you absolutely need to be online, one of these devices will provide you with

Internet access anywhere a reliable mobile phone connection is available.

9 BLUETOOTH MESSAGING APP The newest classification of instant messenger apps, such as FireChat for smartphones, uses bluetooth technology instead of an Internet connection or mobile phone coverage. This allows the phone to be used anywhere, even if networks are down, in a peer-to-peer mode that also helps you discover who is nearby. Coordinate with others in advance so that everyone in a group has the app downloaded before you lose network connectivity for any reason.

164 KEEP YOUR HOME SECURE

"Each man's home is his safest refuge." This 17th-century English legal concept has been interpreted as meaning that you can exclude whomever you wish from your home. To deter criminals, you'll want more than the law on your side.

BE ALARMED Install a burglar alarm with a mix of sensor types, including motion, shock (to detect windows being broken), smoke, heat, and contact sensors.

TAPE IT Install security cameras that record to cloud storage so you'll have evidence if anything happens. You can even view your camera feeds via a smartphone app or Web page if you want to check in on your property remotely.

TRICK THEM You can buy phony alarm company stickers and even fake cameras (which come complete with red LED indicators). Burglars generally make a split-second decision as to whether a target is worth the trouble, so you really don't need to fool them for long.

LIGHT 'EM UP Install a set of motion sensor lights or bright floodlights outside so that no one can hide in the shadows or sneak up to your house.

PRETEND YOU'RE HOME Install timers that turn lights, TVs, and radios on and then off at preprogrammed times to make it appear that you're home.

LOCK UP Don't make it easy; lock all doors and windows when you leave your home. Make sure all entrance doors have a deadbolt lock to better secure against intrusion.

KEEP YOUR KEYS Avoid hiding a key outside; if you do, don't hide it in a flowerpot or other obvious place a burglar might check. Consider asking a trusted neighbor to hold duplicate keys for you instead.

BAR THE DOOR If you have sliding glass doors or windows, install security bars or wooden dowels cut to fit into the tracks so that they can't be popped open. Add decorative reinforcement or kick plates to any entrance door to strengthen it.

WATCH OUT Create or join a neighborhood watch program so that people in your neighborhood will help keep an eye on each other's property.

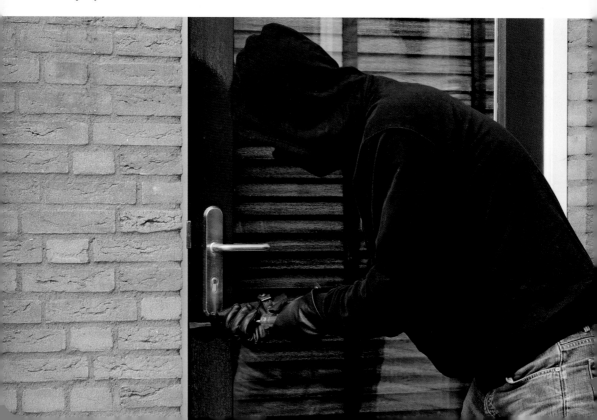

165

STEP UP YOUR SECURITY

If you want to do even more to secure your home, here are some additional tactics to consider. A couple of them may require a little more time or money, but your peace of mind may be worth the cost.

SAY HI Intercom-style doorbells have cameras, speakers, and microphones that connect to your smartphone, so you can answer your door "in person" even if you're away, making it seem like you're home.

GET SPINY To make windows less accessible to intruders, plant thorny bushes or shrubs under them. In addition, keep your lawn mowed and your garden neat—an unkempt yard signals that no one is home.

HIDE IT If you tend to keep any valuables in the house, install a wall safe or other secure secret compartment to hide things from intruders.

BOLT IT If a garage is connected to your house, consider putting an outside accessible deadbolt lock on it, or find some way to physically disable the door with a locked bolt from the inside when you're on vacation for extra protection.

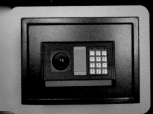

166

LET FIDO HELP OUT

Of course you shouldn't adopt a dog just for protection, but if you're considering making a dog a part of your family anyway, you may find that it can be a great deterrent and early-warning system. Even a tiny lap dog can bark up a storm if it senses an intruder approaching, which can be enough to make the bad guy decide your house is not worth the hassle. If you have one of the larger breeds, you'll also deter burglars who are afraid of dogs.

In fact, just having "Beware of Dog" stickers on windows or signs on gates or fences may deter thieves even if you don't have a dog at home. There are even some alarm systems that play recorded dog barks. All have a deterrent effect but are nowhere near as fun as having an actual four-legged friend.

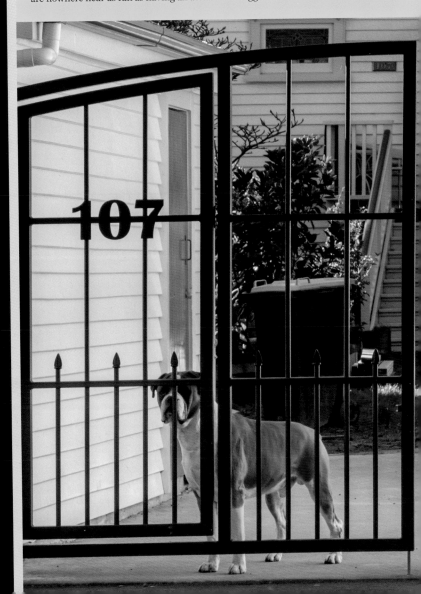

167 HANDLE A HOME INVASION

If you're home when a burglar breaks in or you're the target of a home-invasion-style robbery, you will have to quickly determine how to protect yourself and your family, along with whether you'll be able to protect your property. You never want to risk your own safety or that of others just to protect stuff. Stuff is replaceable but you or your kids are

	1	**2**	**3**
HIDE If your chosen strategy is to hide, then follow these steps to stay safe even if you lose some of your property in the process. This strategy only works before the thief has discovered that you're home.	Be sure all bedrooms have locks on them. That way, if the intruder isn't in your room, you can lock the door. Alternatively, you can have a reinforced panic room to retreat to.	To protect other members of your household that are not yet aware, sneak around and quietly alert them so that they can lock their doors or retreat to the panic room.	If that isn't possible, yell "lock down" to alert them and switch to the **EVADE** strategy.
EVADE If the intruder knows you're home, a strategy of avoiding confrontation can help keep you safe.	If the person is not in your room, lock the door or head to the panic room. If you can't notify everyone quietly then call out "lock down" so everyone can take immediate action to protect themselves.	Call the police and stay on the line until they arrive, if possible.	To attract attention and possibly scare away the thief, set off your car alarm remotely, trigger your home's security alarm, or yell out the window to your neighbors for help.
FLEE If you have a clear exit available, flight may be the wisest strategy	If you attempt to flee and can't for some reason, be ready to switch to either the **EVADE** or **FIGHT** strategies.	If possible, grab your wallet, purse, cell phone, and car keys.	Call the police if you have your cell phone or ask a neighbor to call for you.
FIGHT Sometimes you will have no choice but to fight to protect you and your loved ones. Be mentally and physically prepared to take defend yourself.	Call the police and after they let you know that help is on the way put the phone down without hanging up so the dispatcher can hear what's happening.	Assess what weapons the intruder has. If they have a gun and you don't, or the odds are against you, consider switching to either the **EVADE** or **FLEE** strategies.	When you are first confronted by the intruder, tell them "the police have been called" on the off chance that this will be enough to make them leave.

not. You should plan for each option as a household, and discuss them so that everyone knows the game plan. Your basic options are to hide, evade, flee, or fight. Be prepared to change plans as the circumstances change.

4	5	6
Call the police and stay on the line until they arrive.	Position yourself and others in the corner opposite of the door and prepare to **FIGHT** if the intruder breaks into the room.	Wait for the police to thoroughly clear your house of any unwanted guests.
Be prepared to **FLEE** the room you're in if the intruder confronts you.	If the intruder demands property such as cash, jewelry, and other valuables, comply but keep your distance and be ready to switch to the **FIGHT** strategy if they endanger you or another family member.	Hold out until the police arrive.
If you're not able to get to your car safely to flee, go to a neighbor's house, pound on their door and yell for help. If they don't answer quickly, go to the next house and do the same. If you happen to alert more neighbors in the process, that's not a bad thing.	If no one answers their door, keep fleeing until you are in a safe public place. Ask a bystander to call the police if you don't have your phone with you.	Have the police fully clear your home of any intruders before you enter.
If you have children in the home, have them **FLEE** while you fight to incapacitate the intruder.	If you are armed and the burglar is not, allow them to leave if you can't safely hold them until police arrives	Fight to eliminate the threat. Once the intruder is subdued, hold them until police arrive or use the opportunity to **FLEE**.

168
USE FORCE JUDICIOUSLY

There are times when it's unavoidable to have to use a weapon against someone threatening you, but those times are very few and far between. It's been all too common for a gun owner to panic and injure or kill an innocent person whom they mistook for a threat. In many jurisdictions, you can only use deadly force when you fear for your life and retreat is not possible, or when protecting the life of another. Deadly force used only in defense of property may result in your arrest, a public trial, and prison time. Check with local and state laws to ensure you understand how this may apply to your self-defense. Your first option should always be to avoid confrontation or, if that's unavoidable, to try to diffuse tensions nonviolently.

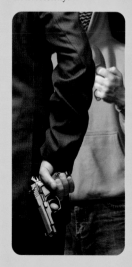

169 INSTALL SMOKE DETECTORS

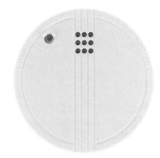

In the event of a house fire, an early warning can often quite literally make the difference between life and death. You should have at least one smoke alarm in every room of your house, except for bathrooms and closets.

SAVE THE DATE Before mounting your smoke detector, write down the date of purchase on the inside of the battery door. After 10 years, replace it.

MOUNT IT HIGH Smoke rises, so mount your detector on the ceiling away from windows and doors and a minimum of 4 inches (10 cm) from any wall. Avoid placing one in the path of heat or steam coming from the kitchen or bathroom; otherwise it may set off false alarms.

MOUNT IT RIGHT All smoke detectors come with a set of specific mounting instructions. Luckily, most make it easy for you, requiring little more than a screwdriver and two screws.

TEST IT OFTEN You should check your detector once a month to ensure that it's working properly. Simply push the button until you hear a loud noise that confirms all is well. If there's no sound, you've got a dud—replace it.

KEEP BATTERIES FRESH Replace the battery once a year. If it starts making an annoying chirping sound, that's your cue that it's time for new juice.

170 DETECT CARBON MONOXIDE

Carbon monoxide (CO) is colorless, tasteless, and odorless—unlike smoke from a fire—which means that the only way to detect it in your home is with a warning device. It's possible to buy combined CO/smoke detectors, but if you don't have the combo version, your CO alarm will *not* also serve as a smoke alarm. In other words, be sure you're covered on both fronts.

Carbon monoxide is produced from incomplete combustion of fossil fuels. Inside the home, CO can be formed by multiple sources such as open flames, space heaters, water heaters, blocked chimneys, or running a car inside a garage. The best practice is to make sure there's at least one CO alarm in every bedroom of your house and at least one on each level, including the basement and garage, and excluding bathrooms and closets. A CO detector should not be placed within fifteen feet of heating or cooking appliances or near any very humid areas such as bathrooms or showers.

SAVE THE DATE Before mounting your CO detector, write the date of purchase on the back. After 5 or 6 years, replace it with a new one.

KEEP IT DOWN Mount at about knee height or a bit higher if you have pets or kids that may knock them off the wall.

PLUG IT IN Many CO detectors are designed to be plugged into an outlet, which makes mounting as simple as plugging it in.

TEST IT OFTEN Check once a month that it's still working, and replace the batteries annually or as needed.

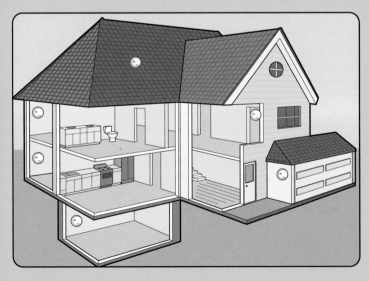

171 PREVENT CARBON MONOXIDE POISONING

If you're snowed in without power, be careful with sources of flame, as these can cause CO poisoning.

PREVENT THE PROBLEM Never bring a charcoal grill or gas generator indoors for any reason. Even using a propane lantern or stove indoors can raise the CO concentration to a dangerous level. Space heaters are also notorious killers, especially if they're left running after everyone goes to bed.

KNOW THE SYMPTOMS Watch for vertigo, fatigue, headaches, or erratic behavior. If more than one person in the house is experiencing these symptoms, it's time to take action.

EVACUATE If you suspect that someone has been affected, get everyone outdoors immediately and open windows and doors to allow ventilation. For mild cases, fresh air is sufficient treatment. For serious cases, seek medical help.

FIND THE PROBLEM Discover the cause of the high concentration of CO and have the situation remedied. Call the fire department for assistance in re-entering your home safely.

173
USE A FIRE EXTINGUISHER

You want to be sure you know how to use your fire extinguisher before you need to. Read the instructions that came with the fire extinguisher, and remember the mnemonic PASS: Pull, Aim, Squeeze, and Sweep.

PULL the pin out of the extinguisher's handle and lever.

AIM the nozzle toward the base of the flames, not at the flames themselves.

SQUEEZE the handle and the lever together to begin spraying the contents of the extinguisher.

SWEEP the nozzle from side to side, moving closer once the fire starts to diminish, until the fire is fully put out. Depending on its size you have about 10 to 20 seconds of operating time before the extinguisher is empty.

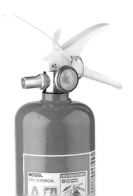

174
FIGHT A FIRE RIGHT

Different types of fires will need to be fought in different ways. In order to extinguish any given blaze safely, you should know the best methods for fighting each class of fire (especially those that are most likely to happen in your home) and always have the correct extinguishers on hand.

CLASS	FIRE TYPE	SAFETY NOTES
A	Common combustibles (wood, paper, clothing, certain plastics)	Use water or smother flames; a foam or CO_2 extinguisher can also work.
B	Flammable liquids and gasses (motor oil, gasoline, common solvents)	Water can spread these fires; spray a foam or CO_2 extinguisher or smother with a wet blanket.
C	Electrical (live electrical equipment and wall outlets)	Never use water, which conducts electricity; use a CO_2 or dry chemical extinguisher.
D	Combustible metals (magnesium, lithium, titanium, and others)	Use a special dry powder chemical extinguisher (there are different types for use on specific metals).
K	Kitchen fires (grease, oils, and fats)	Water can spread these fires; smother with baking soda or use a kitchen extinguisher.

175
KNOW WHEN TO FLEE

176 CLIMB TO SAFETY

If you live in a multistory single-family home or an apartment building that doesn't have fire escapes, it's crucial to have a way to escape if your stairs or front door are blocked by fire and there are no other ways out. You don't want to have to wait for the fire department to bring a ladder to you, since you may be overcome by smoke before they arrive.

Thankfully a number of manufacturers sell emergency ladders that roll or fold to a very small size for easy storage. When you need the ladder, you quickly unfurl it, hook it over a windowsill, and climb to safety. You should have one on each floor; the best practice is to have one for each bedroom. Make sure children in your household know how to use them and review how to use them, when you do your annual fire drill.

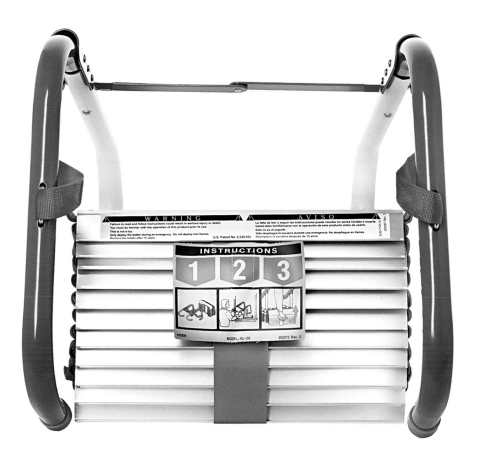

177 DON'T GET SMOKED

Wildfires, a house fire, or even a festive bonfire can expose you to harmful levels of smoke. Hot smoke in particular can be the most dangerous, as it can burn your throat or lungs, and it can also contain other harmful gases.

Signs of smoke inhalation can include coughing; difficulty breathing, hoarse voice or difficulty speaking, nausea or vomiting, headache, or feeling sleepy, disoriented, or confused. If you notice someone with any combination of these symptoms, get them out into fresh air and call emergency responders for help.

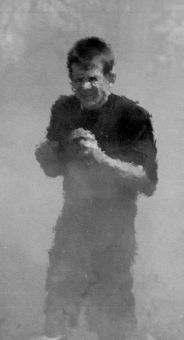

178 STOP, DROP, AND ROLL

What do you do if your clothing catches on fire and there's no fire extinguisher or water source nearby? Your answer is simple and effective: Stop, drop, and roll. Be sure that any kids in your household know this technique, and review it annually as part of any fire drills you conduct for the family (and yes, you really should be doing those fire drills). If you see someone else on fire, yell "Stop, drop, and roll!" at them. They will likely be panicked, so you may need to repeat it a couple of times. You can also help smother the fire but be sure to smother towards their feet so as to not push the flames up to their face.

STOP Be sure you're away from the source of the fire and on a surface you can roll around on. Any unneeded movement will fan the flames and thus increase your chances of being burned by them.

DROP Lay down on the ground while covering your eyes, nose, and mouth with your hands.

ROLL Roll over and back and forth until the flames are out. Remove any burned clothing immediately.

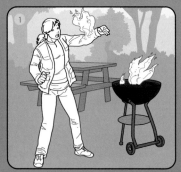
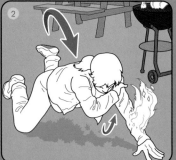
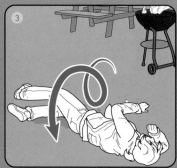

179 ESCAPE A BURNING HOUSE

The key to surviving a fire in your home is having an effective plan in place before the smoldering starts.

KNOW WHERE TO GO Visibility is nearly zero in smoky conditions, so you need to know your escape route by heart. For rooms that have more than one exit, consider which of them would work best in different situations. Practice evacuating with a blindfold on, with someone watching you to keep you safe.

STAY LOW Heat rises; so do smoke and flame. If you're exiting a burning building, get on your hands and knees and crawl toward the nearest safe exit. Cover your mouth and nose with a damp cloth to fight smoke inhalation.

ANTICIPATE Before you open a door, feel for heat on the flat surface rather than the doorknob, which could be dangerously hot. Look under the door, too, for visible flames. If there's any doubt, head to a secondary exit.

SHUN STAIRS If you're trapped on an upper level, get out through a window (have escape ladders at the ready for just such an emergency). Don't use a stairway, because it can act like a chimney, funneling heat and smoke upward.

DON'T BE A HERO Under no circumstance should you remain inside to fight a blaze. If an initial flare-up is not immediately contained, evacuate right away. Run outside, call 911, and let the fire department put out the flames.

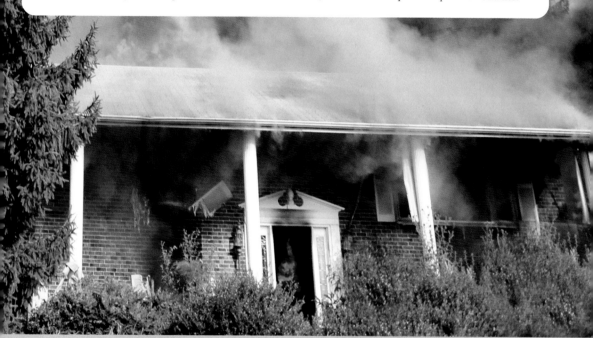

180 SMOTHER A FIRE

Fires need three things to thrive: heat, air, and fuel. Take away any one of these and the fire will go out. An effective way to extinguish a small fire is to deny it air. Use a heavy blanket or coat to completely cover the fire, and press down forcefully. Don't toss it lightly on the flames or it will actually feed the fire. If a pan on the stove ignites, smother it with a metal lid.

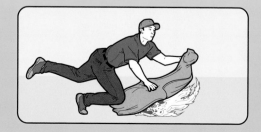

181 RESPOND TO FIRES

If a fire should break out in or near your home, it pays to be well prepared with multiple methods of putting out the fire or getting away from it. Here's a list of good suggestions for your house.

PREPARED

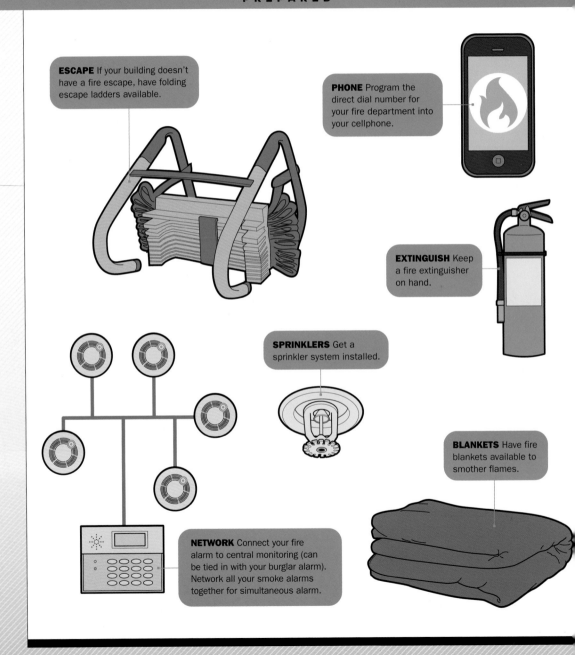

ESCAPE If your building doesn't have a fire escape, have folding escape ladders available.

PHONE Program the direct dial number for your fire department into your cellphone.

EXTINGUISH Keep a fire extinguisher on hand.

SPRINKLERS Get a sprinkler system installed.

BLANKETS Have fire blankets available to smother flames.

NETWORK Connect your fire alarm to central monitoring (can be tied in with your burglar alarm). Network all your smoke alarms together for simultaneous alarm.

Even if you don't have a full fire-fighting plan for your home or if you are somewhere that lacks the resources, you can still deal with fires if you act quickly. Here are some ways to do so.

IMPROVISED

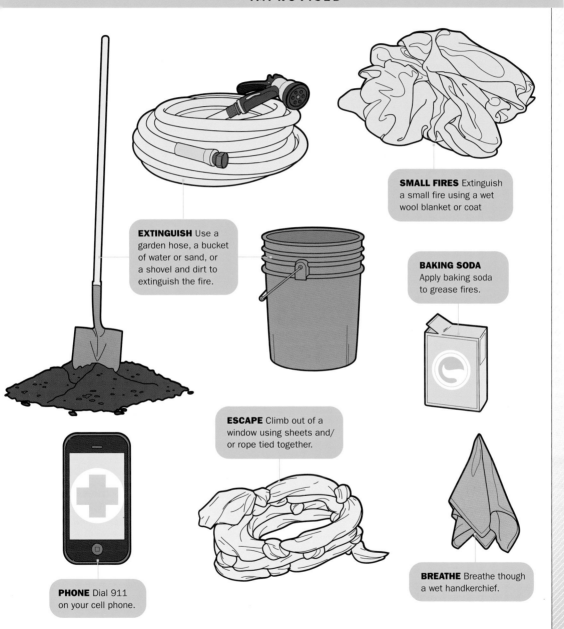

SMALL FIRES Extinguish a small fire using a wet wool blanket or coat

EXTINGUISH Use a garden hose, a bucket of water or sand, or a shovel and dirt to extinguish the fire.

BAKING SODA Apply baking soda to grease fires.

ESCAPE Climb out of a window using sheets and/ or rope tied together.

BREATHE Breathe though a wet handkerchief.

PHONE Dial 911 on your cell phone.

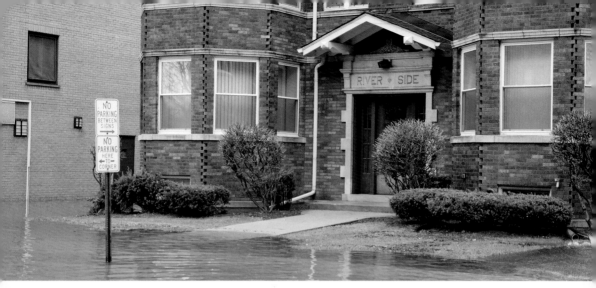

182 FIX A FLOODED BASEMENT

There are many reasons your basement can flood, including burst pipes, rain, broken gutters, leaky windows, a damaged foundation, construction, even tree roots growing into your pipes and blocking them. Even a small amount of water can damage the flooring and anything you've placed on it. If the water level rises higher, items on shelves and in cabinets can be affected. In addition, if your water heater or furnace is in the basement, it can also sustain damage.

A flooded basement is not only an expensive hassle, it's also potentially fatal. If there is any standing water, assume that it's now a dangerous electrical hazard. Before venturing in, make sure that it's safe by having an electrician, a utility employee, or a firefighter turn off the power at the meter (this is much safer than just turning off circuits, but must be done by a professional).

If you have any gas appliances installed in the basement,

be sure to shut off the gas main until the entire basement has been cleared of water.

Once it's safe to enter the basement, the easiest way to drain it is to rent a pump or to have a service do it for you. There will likely be extensive property damage, and the risk of developing mold means that you will need to properly dehumidify and rehabilitate the space. This can be complex, time consuming, and expensive. If you do not possess the experience to handle it right, hire professionals who do.

To prevent or limit damage, protect your belongings by placing them on shelves in watertight containers. Install a sump pump; if you live in a particularly damp area, run a dehumidifier in the basement during the cold and damp months. Install any electrical outlets and equipment high up. Install ground fault interrupter (GFI) outlets as required by code, and don't leave extension cords on the floor.

183 BUILD A WALL

Sandbags will not create a perfectly waterproof seal, but placed correctly they are quite effective at diverting relatively slow-moving water so that it runs around rather than through your home. Before building your wall, think about how you'd remove any water that might get trapped between the wall and your home. (Do you have a pump? Would you have to bail it out

by hand?). Place a bag over any floor drains to stop gray water or sewage from backing up if local sewer lines get overloaded. Most experts say not to stack the bags more than three layers high (about 1 foot (30 cm)). If waters are rising higher than that, you should probably evacuate rather than trying to fend off increasingly dangerous floodwaters.

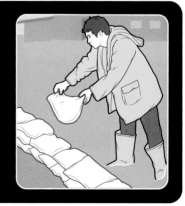

184 MAKE A PYRAMID

Pyramids made from sandbags are used to reinforce levees or as free-standing walls, and can be built much higher with successive layers.

STEP 1 Place sandbags with the untied opening in the direction that the water is expect to flow from. Tuck the open end under itself to anchor the flap under the bag's weight.

STEP 2 Finish laying out your entire first row.

STEP 3 Lay a second row on the ground next to the first. Offset the second row so that the center of each second-row bag is positioned adjacent to the space between the first-row bags.

STEP 4 Lay a third row next to the first two and offset once again.

STEP 5 Start out your second layer by placing a bag offset on top and between the first and second row.

STEP 6 Lay another row next to that, on top and between the second and third row.

STEP 7 Continue stacking bags in this fashion until your pyramid is up to the height you desire.

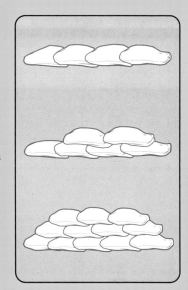

185 FILL SANDBAGS CORRECTLY

Manually filling, moving, and placing sandbags can be physically demanding work. Because this involves repeatedly lifting and carrying heavy sandbags it's best done in small groups of four people, but it can be done with less people if need be. Each person in a group should have a role. The key roles are bagger, shoveler, and mover. If you have a fourth person, they can rotate into the other three positions as well as help out with moving filled bags or whatever needs support to keep the process going.

Both burlap and poly bags are used to make sandbags. Both will last about eight months to a year before needing to be replaced. Sandbags filled one-half to two-thirds full should generally be left untied. Tied bags, filled slightly fuller, are mostly used for specific purposes such as filling holes or holding objects in position. Bags should also be tied shut if you're transporting or stockpiling them. However, since they are often filled at or near the placement site, tying the bags is frequently a waste of time and effort.

STEP 1 Make sure everyone is wearing work gloves, especially the person serving as a bagger, since their hands can be injured by the shovel during filling.

STEP 2 The bagger crouches with their feet apart and arms extended, placing the bottom of the empty bag on the ground.

STEP 3 Next, the bagger folds the open end of the bag outward a few inches to form a collar and holds the bag open.

STEP 4 The shoveler carefully places sand into the bag.

STEP 5 Finally, the mover adds the bag to the wall.

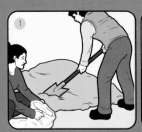
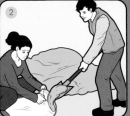
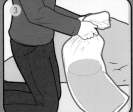
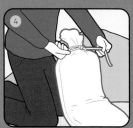

186 GET KIDS READY

Helping kids prepare for emergencies can be scary for them. But emergencies can strike anyone at any time, and the best defense is preparation. Reassuring kids that planning and preparing allows everyone to better handle the problem can help them cope. Here are some age-appropriate activities to help kids prepare.

ELEMENTARY SCHOOL AGE

- Conduct a scavenger hunt for items that should go into an emergency kit.
- Volunteer to take part in a food drive or other community preparedness activity.
- Discuss different places where emergencies could happen (such as at school, at home, or at a park) and how to prepare for those different types of situations.
- Have children write and illustrate a storybook on how to prepare for an emergency.
- Ask them questions such as: What do we do when a tornado comes? What is an emergency plan? Where is our emergency kit? What do we put into it?
- Work together to make a mini disaster kit and go bag for each child; include a few fun toys and something else that provides them comfort, like a stuffed animal.

JUNIOR HIGH SCHOOL AGE

- Take a first-aid or CPR class.
- Teach them how to shut off the utilities in case of emergency.
- Have them write a report, create a poster, or make a short video about a specific hazard.
- Tour a fire department or other emergency service provider.
- Take a class to get licensed for HAM radio.
- Work together to create an everyday carry kit.

HIGH SCHOOL AGE

- Volunteer with the Red Cross, a local CERT (Community Emergency Response Team) program, or a fire department explorer program.
- Create an emergency kit for their car.
- Have them write an article for their school newspaper or blog or do a school assignment on emergency preparedness.
- Brainstorm how they could work with a local disaster relief organization to prepare others for an emergency, and then make it happen.
- Teach them how to purify water with bleach, by boiling, or with other water-purification techniques.

187 EXPLAIN CLEARLY

As a parent you want to protect your children during a disaster. You may not want to discuss the situation in front of them, or let them see how worried you are, but avoiding the issue might be equally stressful for them. Listen to your kids and ask them about their feelings. Give an appropriate amount of detail for them to understand the situation.

Repetitive media coverage can increase concerns or anxiety; consider watching with your children so you can talk with them and answer questions in the moment. Discuss next steps for the family, and involve them in the decision-making process. Review and update family disaster and communication plans.

Also, seek support from counseling, friends, or family to help with your own stress; you'll be better able to support your kids.

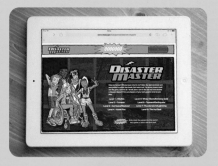

188 PREPARE ONLINE

A wide variety of preparedness activities can be done online at various websites, or in the form of downloadable content such as coloring books, comic books, and games that are fun and engaging for kids. Google for a resource you like or try some of these favorites:

- *Disaster Master*
- *Kids Get a Plan*
- *Preparedness 101: Zombie Pandemic*
- *Mickey & Friends: Disaster Preparedness Activity Book*

189 TEACH YOUR KIDS TO BE SAFE

There are a few skills every child should learn to help keep them safe when you're not there to protect or guide them.

DON'T WANDER Lost children become scared very quickly, and their natural response is to begin searching for their family. Remind your children to stop as soon as they realize they are lost and to call for help with their cell phone or a whistle. Assure them that staying in one place allows them to be found more easily.

STAY SAFE AT HOME Very young children don't have the judgment to correctly assess if it's okay to open the door for someone. It might be a friendly neighbor but it could also be someone with ill intentions. Instruct them to not answer the door for anyone, and to keep all the doors and windows closed and locked. Additionally, you can install a video doorbell that routes the video signal to your smartphone so that you can see who is at your door and interact with them through the intercom even when you're away from home.

CALL FOR HELP As soon as they are able, kids should learn how to dial 911 and report an emergency. Spend time with them to regularly review how to make emergency phone calls, teaching your children to say their name, address, and the type of emergency such as a fire or that someone is sick. Remind them to follow the dispatcher's instructions, and then stay on the line until help does arrive, to open the door when the dispatcher tells them to, and to turn on outdoor lights if it's nighttime.

TRUST YOUR FEELINGS This one skill can help your child avoid many potentially dangerous situation. The concept is simple: When a child feels uncomfortable in any situation, they should find an adult that they can trust, such as a police officer, a teacher, or instead to head home. If they have a cell phone, they can call a parent or emergency number. Tell them it's better to ask for help, and that if it turns out to be nothing you won't be mad at them for doing the right thing. In other words, better safe than sorry.

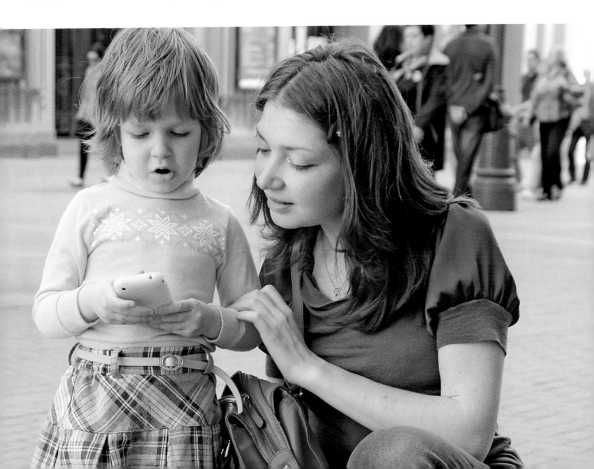

190 SPOT A POTENTIAL RUNAWAY

Every at-risk child will display different signs that they might be planning to run away. Here are some things to keep an eye out for.

Worrisome changes in behavior can include a variety of emotional or mental health–related issues, including overeating, loss of appetite, sleeping all day, insomnia, staying away from home, avoiding family members, or never wanting to leave their room. Teens may also have mood swings or other signs of stress.

It's normal for teenagers to be rebellious, but some behaviors may actually be a precursor to running away. Be concerned about poor performance in school, bad grades, truancy, breaking rules at home, refusing to do chores, or picking fights.

A more obvious sign is a child threatening or hinting that they will run away. Other members of the family may hear rumors through friends, school, or even other parents that their child is thinking of leaving.

To survive as a runaway, your child will need money and resources. Some prepare by making withdrawals from their bank accounts or looking for other ways to gather cash or valuable. They may also pack a bag of clothes and personal effects so that they can leave at a moment's notice.

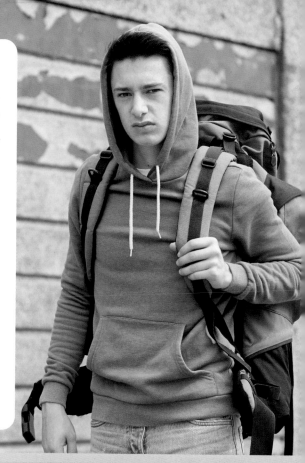

191 CONVINCE A TEEN TO STAY

If you're facing the moment when a teen is threatening to leave, it's time to switch tactics to see if you can persuade them to stay. Kids often leave home after an argument with their parents or after some major event, but below are four tactics to try *before* they leave.

CALM THINGS DOWN Try to get your child to calm down for a few minutes. Say something like "Why don't you sit right here in the kitchen and have a snack before you leave. I'll be back in five minutes." It's not a good idea to send the kid to their room; they may have all their supplies there and might bolt more readily.

ASK QUESTIONS Ask them about the situation, but don't focus on what they are feeling because some kids want to argue about how they're feeling rather than discuss the real issue. Try asking, "What's going on?" or "What happened to make you want to leave?"

BE PERSUASIVE Teens may be running away from problems they can't handle or because they are feeling overwhelmed. Ask your child questions like "What's so different about this situation that you think you can't handle it?" Remind them that things will eventually be ok, that "facing the music" is part of life and that you've had similar challenges. Convince them you believe in their ability to cope with this and the even if they made a mistake, it's not the end of the world. By not blaming them, you may be able to have an environment that allows them to feel okay with staying.

BE FRANK Calmly let your child know that you're concerned about them and that you're afraid they might run away from home. Suggest that they find someone to talk about what's bothering them and be supportive of finding positive ways of help them cope with their stress. Let them know that you don't want them to run away and that you're committed to helping the family work things out.

192 HANDLE A MISSING TEEN

If, despite your best efforts to convince your teen not to run away, they manage to do so anyway, here are some steps to help find them. Law enforcement may offer some additional support or suggestions. No matter what happens, this will be an emotional time, and you'll likely experience a gamut of feelings, including anger, fear, and shame.

Immediately notify the police and file a missing persons report, as there is no waiting period for reporting children under age 18. Call the National Runaway Safeline (NRS) at 1-800-RUNAWAY; NRS runs a 24-hour confidential hotline for teens and their families, and you can leave a message with them for your child.

Search their room for anything that may give you a clue as to where they went. Look at phone bills, e-mail activity, text messages, credit card activity, bank statements, and other records for clues where your child might have gone.

Reach out and get support from other family members, trusted friends, or other members of your support network during and after the ordeal. Some children will head to a nearby friend or relative for refuge. Call anyone you think your child might reach out to, and ask them to let you know if they contacted them. Or, ask that person to tell your child to call the NRS to receive or leave messages if you suspect that your child doesn't want to call you directly.

Print posters in case your teen is still in the area. Contact the news desk of your local television station or newspaper. Also, call your child's school. Talk to the staff, teachers, or counselors for any information that might be useful.

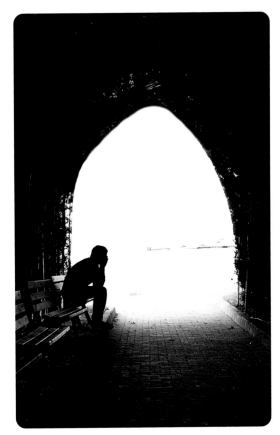

193 HELP A LOST CHILD

If you happen to come across a young lost child in a park, store, or other public place, you can do the right thing by helping them get reunited with their parents.

STEP 1 Get down to the child's level. Crouch or sit with them to establish rapport.

STEP 2 Ask if they need help. Don't assume anything— the child may be fine, so be sure help is needed.

STEP 3 If they say yes, assure them you'll help them and stay with them.

STEP 4 Gather any information they are able to tell about their parents, such as their names, the clothing that they

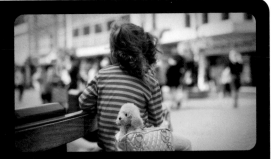

are wearing, and what they look like. Ask if they know a parent's phone number.

STEP 5 Contact police, security, or any available staff for assistance.

STEP 6 Stay at the location where you found the child.

194 CHILDPROOF YOUR HOME

Accidents, especially with kids, occur quickly and without warning. All it takes is that one distracted moment for an injury to occur to a child, but these little emergencies can be prevented with a little bit of effort. It might help to crawl around your house on your hands and knees to see things from their perspective. Here are some tips to help make your home safe for kids.

AROUND THE HOUSE

- ☐ Keep floors and lower shelves free of small items that could present a choking hazard.
- ☐ Check to see if any plants in the house are potentially poisonous.
- ☐ Keep potpourri and any flower arrangements with rocks or marbles out of reach.
- ☐ Cover unused electrical outlets with outlet protectors or safety caps.
- ☐ Secure rugs to the floors or fit them with anti-slip pads.
- ☐ Install finger-pinch guards on doors.
- ☐ Attach TVs, equipment, bookshelves and other furniture to the wall with secure brackets, especially in earthquake country.
- ☐ Install stops on all removable drawers.
- ☐ Make sure any room near a water source, such as a bathroom or kitchen, has ground-fault interrupter (GFI) outlets installed.
- ☐ Secure gas fireplaces with a valve cover or key.
- ☐ Install screens on working fireplaces.
- ☐ Tie window-blind cords out of kids' reach to prevent strangulation.
- ☐ Use safety gates at the top and bottom of stairs and in the doorways of rooms with hazards, such as kitchens.

BATHROOM

- ☐ Keep cosmetics, razors, grooming scissors, and medicines or vitamins out of reach or locked up.
- ☐ Hide wastebasket under the sink or in a locked cabinet, or ensure it has a secure lid.
- ☐ Install childproof latches installed on all cabinet doors.
- ☐ Store medicines and other products in their original containers.
- ☐ Keep all hair dryers, curling irons, and electric razors unplugged when not in use.
- ☐ Install nonskid strips in bathtubs and showers.

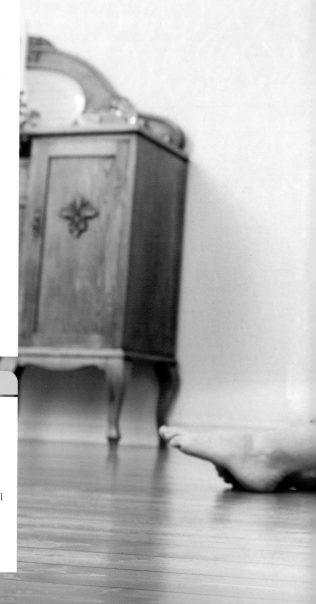

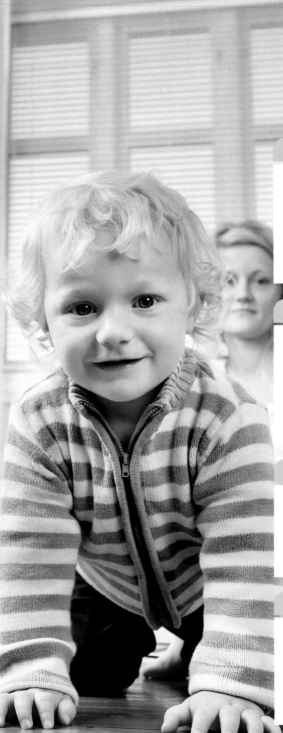

KITCHEN

☐ Keep knives, forks, scissors, and other sharp tools in a drawer with a childproof latch.
☐ Keep bottles containing alcohol stored out of reach.
☐ Install childproof latches installed on all cabinet doors.
☐ Turn pot handles away from the front of the stove to prevent accidents or spills.

HOME OFFICE/WORKSPACE

☐ Keep scissors and office supplies where your child can't grab them.
☐ Hang a mirror on the wall above workstations or computer monitors so you can see kids playing in the area behind you.
☐ Keep any hazardous tools, poisons, or chemical products in your immediate control when in use.

SAFE STORAGE

☐ Store matches and lighters securely.
☐ Store any toxic or poisonous substances in their original containers, and out of reach and sight.
☐ Store firearms unloaded in a locked case with ammunition securely stored in a separate place.

OUTDOORS

☐ Keep garages and garden sheds locked to prevent access to tools and chemicals.
☐ Ensure walkways and outdoor stairways are well lit.
☐ Make sure pools, even shallow wading or decorative pools, are fenced off with a self-closing gate and a childproof lock.

195 DON'T HAVE A HOT DOG

Some pet owners don't realize that, even with the windows slightly open, the temperature inside of a car rises pretty quickly. It some circumstances the interior temperature can increase by 50 °F (122 °C) in about an hour. Lowering the windows just a little bit doesn't cool things down very much.

Signs of heat stroke in a dog include excessive panting or drooling, difficulty breathing, rapid pulse, disorientation, collapse, and unconsciousness. Heat stroke can also lead to seizure and respiratory arrest.

If you see a dog in a car on a hot day, it may be hard for you to know if it's okay. If you're worried, here are steps to take to help.

STEP 1 Note the car's color, model, make, license plate number, specific location, and time you first observed the car. Additionally, write down your observations of the dog's condition, especially if it's displaying any signs of distress. This will be helpful to any emergency responders who might get involved later.

STEP 2 If the pet doesn't appear to be in distress, and if there are businesses nearby, find a store employee or a security guard and ask them to make an announcement to try and find the car's owner.

STEP 3 If all else fails, contact animal control or call your local emergency number to request help for the animal.

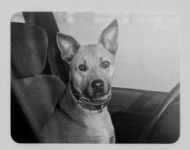

196 GIVE THE RIGHT MEDICINES

Is it safe to give drugs intended for human use to your pets? The answer is, "Maybe." Some drugs will be toxic to pets, and human-size doses will be dangerous for smaller animals. Therefore, you should always consult your veterinarian for advice before giving them any medication. Here are some drugs that you might be able to use with your pet in an emergency.

DRUG	ANIMAL USE	CATS	DOGS
IBUPROFEN OR NAPROXEN	N/A	Toxic at any dose	Toxic at any dose
BUFFERED OR ENTERIC-COATED ASPIRIN	Inflammation and pain	Unsafe	OK
ACETAMINOPHEN (TYLENOL)	Fever and pain	Fatal	OK with proper dose*
DIPHENHYDRAMINE (BENADRYL)	Allergies and motion sickness	Injected	OK
FAMOTIDINE (PEPCID AC), CIMETIDINE (TAGAMET HB), RANITIDINE (ZANTAC)	Acid reflux, *Helicobacter pylori* infection, inflammatory bowel disease, canine parvovirus, ulcers	OK	OK
DIMENHYDRINATE (DRAMAMINE)	Motion sickness	OK	OK
LOPERAMIDE (IMODIUM)	Diarrhea	OK	OK
BISMUTH SUBSALICYLATE (KAOPECTATE)	Diarrhea	Fatal	OK
CETIRIZINE (ZYRTEC)	Allergies	OK	OK
LORATADINE (CLARITIN)	Allergies	OK	OK
AMOXICILLIN, AMPICILLIN, TETRACYCLINE	Infection	OK	OK

* ask your vet

197 HANDLE AN INJURED PET

Pets—even the ones who are normally very docile and friendly—can become unpredictable and may bite or scratch you if they're injured or sick. Here are some tips for handling a pet who needs medical help.

KEEP YOUR DISTANCE Keep your face far enough away from their mouth that you're not an easy target for a bite.

MUZZLE THEM If your pet isn't vomiting, muzzling them will allow you to more easily and safely handle them while taking them to the veterinarian for treatment.

WRAP THEM UP Take a towel or blanket and wrap them in it several times. Doing so keeps their legs tucked in and makes it easier to carry them. Some animals may also find this comforting.

CRATE THEM If your pet is crate trained, place them in their crate for transportation.

COVER THEM Use a towel to cover your pet's head; this will often reduce their stress by reducing visual stimuli. Observe your pet and remove the towel if it makes them more nervous.

MOVE CAREFULLY When carrying or driving, do so with care so as to not to jostle or scare your pet.

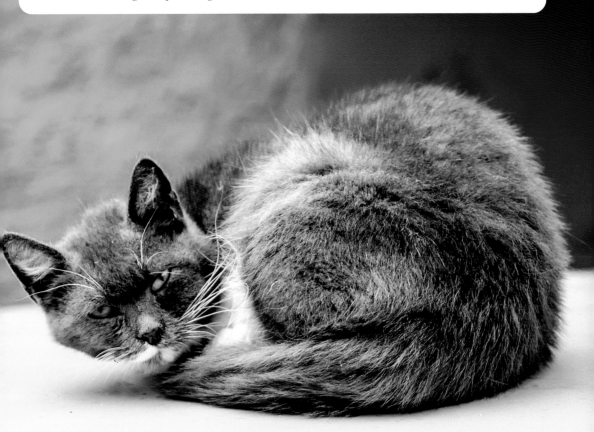

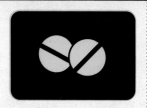
198 GIVE A PET CPR

CPR for cats and dogs is similar to human CPR but, like any skill, it still requires training and practice to do effectively.

STEP 1 Open the animal's mouth to make sure their airway is clear. If they are choking on an object, see if you can reach in with your fingers and carefully remove it. Be quick when doing so, to avoid being bitten. If the pet in question is unconscious and not breathing, you need to start CPR.

STEP 2 Lay your unconscious pet on their right side, lift the head to align with the neck, open the mouth, and then pull the tongue forward. Use some cloth, such as your shirtsleeve, to grab the tongue more easily. Look, listen, or feel for breathing. If there are no signs of breathing, start performing rescue breathing. Give four to five rescue breaths by firmly holding their snout and blowing just enough air though the nose for the chest to rise. For smaller dogs and cats, your mouth will go around both the mouth and nose.

STEP 3 Feel for a pulse in the femoral artery, high inside the thigh. If there is no pulse, start chest compressions. If possible, have someone help you with CPR as well as with transporting your pet to the vet.

STEP 4 For a dog, find the heart by bringing their left elbow back to their chest. Place the heel of your palm over the heart, intertwine your fingers, and lock your arms. Give 30 chest compressions at a rate of about 80–120 times per minute followed by two rescue breaths. Compress the chest about 2 to 3 inches (5–7.5 cm) for larger dogs and 1/2 to 1 inch (1.25–2.5 cm) for small dogs and cats (squeeze using both hands around the chest in this case). Stop and check for a pulse after five cycles of compressions and rescue breaths.

STEP 5 Continue CPR until it becomes unsafe to continue for any reason or until you become too exhausted to continue, veterinary professionals take over care, or the animal regains a pulse.

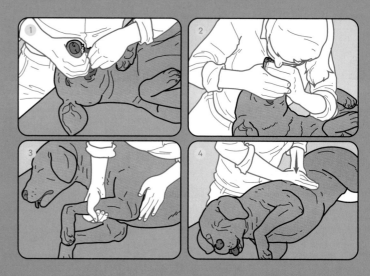

199 RUN OFF A RACCOON

Raccoons can be found living in the crawl space under your house, in the chimney, up in your attic, or just sneaking in through your pet door to feast on your cat's food. They can attack pets or even humans, and are known rabies carriers. Thankfully there are plenty of humane ways to shoo these furry bandits off, including with bright lights, loud music, and unpleasant scents such as cider vinegar placed in a bowl near places that they frequent around your home.

Next, seal any entrances they might use to get inside. If you encounter a raccoon in one of your rooms, don't try to fight it or scare it away; simply lock up your pets in a safe area, close any doors to keep it out of the rest of the house, and open a window or door to the outside. Eventually it will leave on its own. If you've tried all these measures to no avail, you may need to trap and release the beast, or call in a wildlife removal service to do it for you.

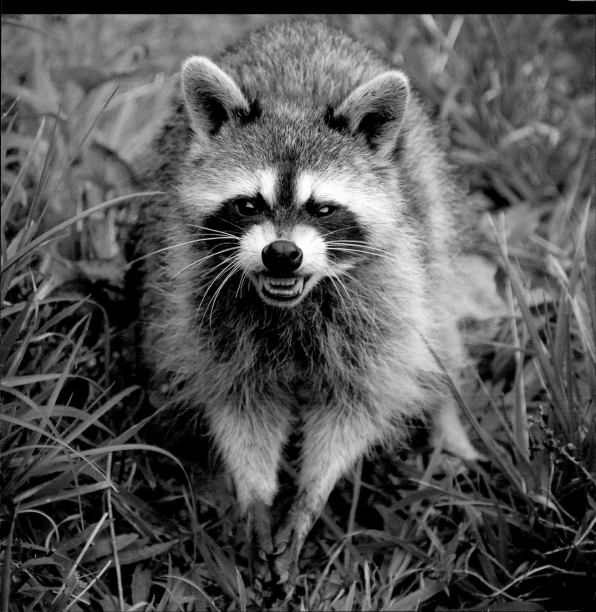

200 KNOW WHEN TO GO TO THE VET

Since animals can't talk, it's hard to know just how sick they are. You'll have to rely on your own experience with your pet to figure out what's different about its behavior or health. If you notice any of these symptoms, it's time to contact your vet for more advice.

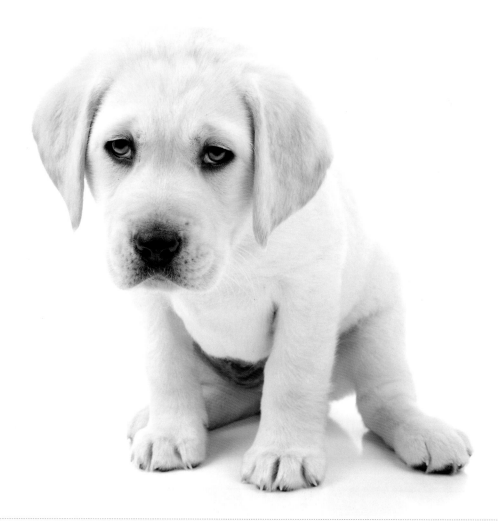

- Difficulty breathing or wheezing
- Discharge from the ears, eyes, nose, or other orifice
- Rapid weight loss
- Loss of appetite
- Lethargy
- Excessive groaning

- Excessive scratching or chewing
- Eye problems (pawing at eyes, squinting, etc.)
- Hot spots or infections
- Limping
- Swelling or bloating
- Unusual odor

- Persistent vomiting
- Bloody stool or urine
- Continuous diarrhea or frequent urination
- Difficulty defecating or urinating
- Very dark and/or thick urine

201 TRANSPORT YOUR PET SAFELY

Unfortunately, ambulances for pets are rare. If you need to get your animal to the veterinarian, you'll often have to do so yourself. For less urgent issues you can simply put the animal in a crate or, for a dog, (and the very rare cat) have them ride in the car as usual. If your animal is very sick or has suffered a traumatic injury, you'll have to take care in transporting them. Avoid carrying animals that are sick or hurt in your arms; even pets that are normally docile may become aggressive when in pain or afraid.

STEP 1 Grab two large towels and a medium-sized towel.

STEP 2 Use a muzzle if you have one available for your own safety unless they are vomiting, coughing, or unconscious.

STEP 3 Spread one large towel out by your pet's back.

STEP 4 Small animals can be safely moved onto the towel by two people. For larger pets, you'll need three: one to hold the head, another for the shoulders, and a third for the hips. Coordinate a gentle slide up onto the towel.

STEP 5 Carefully lift and load your pet into your vehicle. When lifting, use the medium-sized towel to support their head by slinging it under their chin. If possible, have someone ride in the back to help keep them still and calm.

STEP 6 Cover the pet with the third towel to keep them warm and to treat for shock.

STEP 7 Drive slowly and carefully. It's tempting to speed to the vet's office as quickly as possible, but any jostling could further injure your pet.

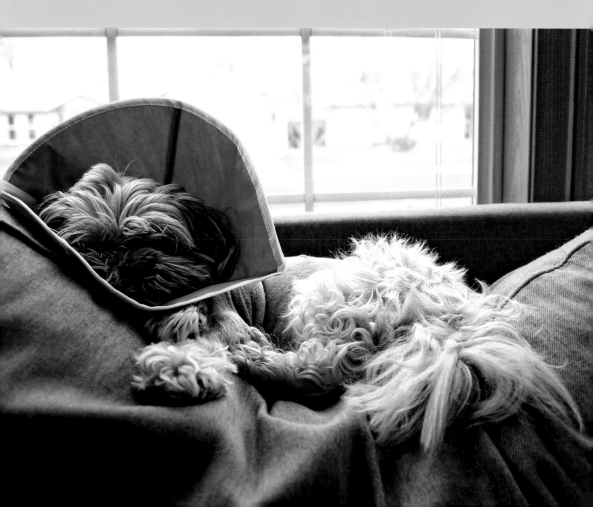

202 AVOID A DOG ATTACK

If you're confronted by an aggressive dog, here are some tactics for handling the situation.

STAY CALM Dogs will react less aggressively to you if you're calm.

AVOID EYE CONTACT Dogs may see this behavior as challenging.

DON'T SMILE Bared teeth are usually an aggression signal among animals.

STAND STILL Even if the dog comes close, it's safer to stand still than to run, which might trigger a predatory response to chase and attack.

DISTRACT THE DOG Offer the dog a stick or other object within reach to chew on. If you have any food, throw it nearby and see if the dog becomes distracted enough for you to get away.

BE ASSERTIVE If none of the quiet approaches is effective in deterring the dog, try commanding it in a deep, confident voice to "go home."

GET UP If the dog seems likely to lunge for you, climb onto a parked car or dumpster.

LEAVE SLOWLY If the dog appears to lose interest, slowly and carefully leave the area.

CALL 911 If you have your phone, call your local emergency number to request help.

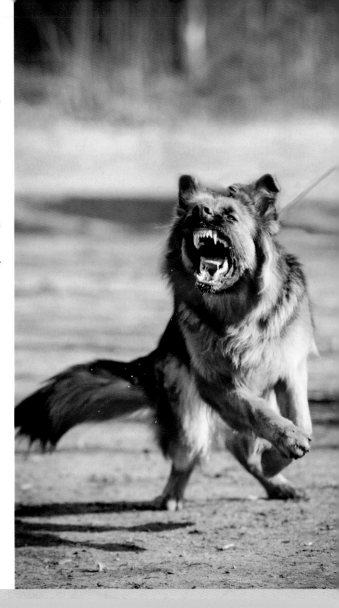

203 UNDERSTAND AGGRESSION

Why do dogs often act aggressively? Entire books have been written about this topic along with the multitude of factors and circumstances that can trigger aggression. Some of the most common causes are the perceived need to show their dominance over a rival and to protect their territory or pack members (which, to a dog, may include its human family).

Dogs may also become aggressive when guarding their food or favorite toys. As far as basic animal instincts, a dog who is in heat or trying to reach another dog in heat may get unusually aggressive. And it's worth remembering that even domesticated dogs still have predatory instincts and may attack small animals or chase someone running from them.

Just like humans, dogs can also react aggressively to fear, frustration, or pain. If unable to escape a stressful situation, they may fight instead of fleeing, or lash out if frustrated by events. If hurt, they may react in an unpredictable fashion, including aggressively. Knowing all of these factors may help you assess whether an animal is likely to attack.

204 RECOGNIZE WARNING SIGNS

Once you know the conditions likely to trigger aggressive behavior in a dog, then you'll want to observe a potentially threatening animal carefully to determine if it's likely to attack. Dogs usually exhibit a set of escalating warning behaviors prior to attacking. The more warning signs you observe, the more cautious you should be around the animal.

Dogs bark in various ways to communicate, but a low, guttural bark is their way of giving a warning or threat. Likewise, growling or snarling are very strong indicators.

Body posture can be another useful indicator. Watch to see if its ears are pulled back, lying flat against the head, or if the dog becomes very still and rigid. They may also lunge forward or charge.

A dog's mouth is one of its primary ways of interacting with the world, so it's not always immediately easy to tell if you're at risk of being bitten. A dog may use its mouth to gently grab someone in order to establish dominance without biting, or push or poke something with its muzzle [A]. If this escalates to light nips [B], get out of the situation before the next possible step of more serious bites causes marks or bruises or even serious injury.

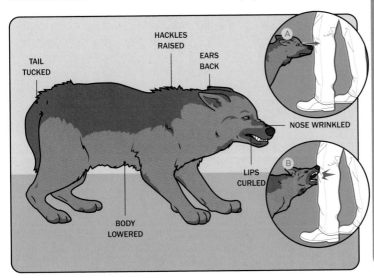

HACKLES RAISED

EARS BACK

TAIL TUCKED

NOSE WRINKLED

LIPS CURLED

BODY LOWERED

205 FIGHT OFF AN ATTACKING DOG

If you've done everything that you can to avoid or get away from an aggressive dog, then you're down to the last option: fight.

If you're attacked, fight back by punching and kicking, along with yelling commands at the dog with significant force. Dog attacks can be deadly, and you should fight for your life with whatever means that you have available. If you happen to carry pepper spray, it can be effective against dogs.

Wrestle the dog using your full body weight to subdue them, and once the dog is subdued, call 911. Beware of the owner, as attacking their dog may create a conflict that can also escalate violently.

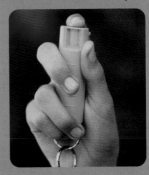

206 TEACH YOUR CHILD DOG SAFETY

Children should learn how to carefully approach and interact with strange dogs to reduce their chance of getting bitten. A few basics: Always ask permission to pet a dog; don't tease dogs (or any animals); and do not disturb a dog with a litter of puppies, as she will be instinctively protective. If a strange dog approaches your child, they should stand still, be quiet,

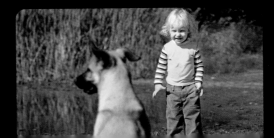

207 READ MSDS

Material safety data sheets (MSDS), now more commonly called safety data sheets (SDS) are not really intended for consumers, but often readily available online. These describe the potential hazards of everything from everyday office supplies such as toner to household cleaners to the chemicals used in manufacturing. As a layperson, you can use an SDS to become more informed about the products you use, as well as learning how to treat someone exposed to the product. This information can be especially useful during a major disaster in which access to regular medical care may be difficult or impossible.

The SDS for each substance includes information on the item's chemical composition, toxicity, and potential health effects of exposure.

Other sections provide detailed guidelines on how to handle any accidents involving the chemical (such as spills, leaks, or explosions), and how to recognize the symptoms of overexposure.

There is also a set of first-aid and emergency response procedures with specific protocols for treating people, objects, or environments exposed to the substance.

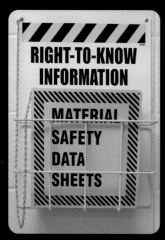

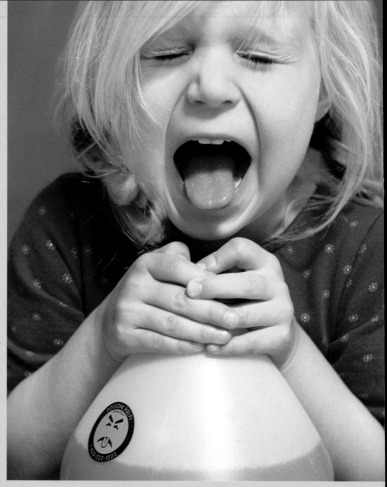

208 MEET MR. YUK

These days, the average kid associates the image of a skull and crossbones more with pirates than with poison. Dr. Richard Moriarty, a pediatrician and founder of the Pittsburgh Poison Center, was concerned that the old symbol didn't effectively communicate to kids that a substance is dangerous to eat or drink. He showed a range of colors to children in day care centers, and this "yucky" green was rated the least appealing. Mr. Yuk has been adopted as the official warning symbol by the National Poison Center Network.

If you have children in your home, place Mr. Yuk stickers on all containers of dangerous household chemicals, even those that are securely stored. Sit down with your children and explain what the sticker means. To request a free sheet of Mr. Yuk stickers, send a self-addressed stamped envelope to:

Mr. Yuk
Pittsburgh Poison Center
200 Lothrop Street
PFG 01-01-01
Pittsburgh,
PA 15213

209 READ THE FIRE DIAMOND

Have you ever noticed one of these placards on the outside of a building? It's a quick reference to the hazards you'll find inside. The NFPA 704 Standard System for the Identification of the Hazards of Materials for Emergency Response, also known as the "fire diamond," provides basic information for emergency personnel responding to a fire or spill and those planning for emergency response.

Each part of the diamond is color-coded to represent a different hazard, with a number representing its severity; the white diamond may contain a code indicating a specific hazard (see below for a list).

If you need to enter an area that's marked with the fire diamond, note whether it has any 3s, 4s, or special hazard markings. If so, be extremely careful. Avoid the area entirely if you're uncertain on how to safely proceed, especially if you notice any leaks, spills, odors, or gas.

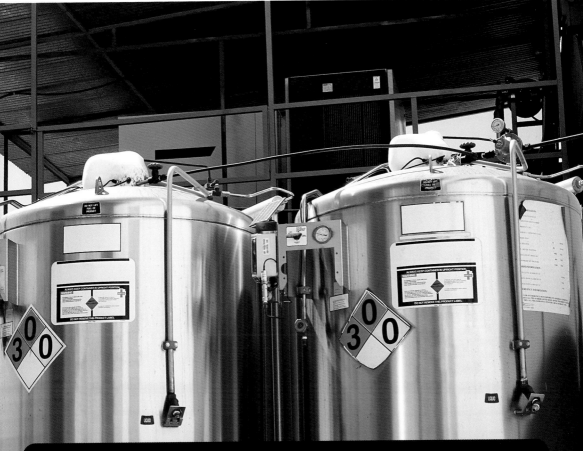

COLORS

BLUE Acute, short-term health hazard

RED Flammable

YELLOW Instability or explosive danger

WHITE Special hazards

NUMBERS

0 No danger

1 Minor hazard

2 Moderate hazard

3 Serious hazard

4 Extreme hazard

CODES

OX Oxidizer (can react with heat and fuel to create fire)

W Reacts with water

SA Simple asphyxiant gas

COR Corrosive

ACID Acidic

ALK Alkaline

BIO Biological hazard

POI Poisonous

RA, RAD Radioactive

CYL, CRYO Cryogenic

210 GET OUT OF A SKID

You may have no warning of a skid until you suddenly lose control and end up heading sideways down the highway. Here's how to regain control.

STEP 1 Resist the temptation to hit the brakes. To steer out of the skid, you need to have tires rolling, not locked up.

STEP 2 It may seem counterintuitive, but turn the steering wheel into the direction of the skid (for example, if your car's right side is moving forward, turn your wheel to the right). Do this gently without overreacting. If your wheels start to skid in the other direction, turn the steering wheel that way. Be ready to straighten the wheel as your vehicle returns to its normal course.

STEP 3 Apply very light pressure on the accelerator to help bring the vehicle back into position.

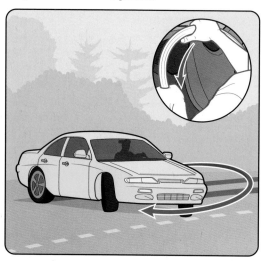

211 STEER WITH BLOWN TIRES

When a tire blows out, it will pull the vehicle in the direction of the flat. This is really scary and can cause you to lose control, but if you stay calm and know what to do, you can steer yourself to safety.

DON'T PANIC Fight the urge to overcorrect or to slam on the brakes, which will cause a skid.

SLOW DOWN Hold the steering wheel firmly, ease off the accelerator, switch on your turn signal, and start moving toward the shoulder of the road.

SIGNAL Once you reach the shoulder, switch on your emergency flasher to warn approaching vehicles.

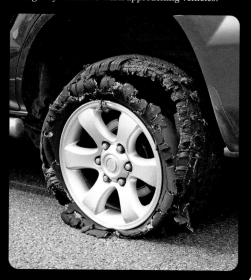

212 DEAL WITH BRAKE FAILURE

You press on the brake pedal and it goes to the floor without slowing the vehicle. Now what? Don't turn off the ignition and remove the key; the steering column will lock. Leave your foot off the accelerator to slow down, and negotiate traffic and turns as best you can. If you're going downhill and picking up speed, shift to a lower gear (even automatic transmissions give you this ability) and gradually apply the emergency brake. If there's an uphill route, take it.

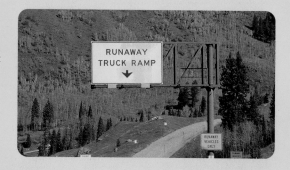

213 DRIVE SAFELY ON FLOODED ROADS

Every year, people lose their lives when their vehicles get washed away as they try to drive on flooded roads.

STUDY THE NUMBERS A measly 6 inches (15 cm) of water will cause most cars to lose control and possibly stall. Double that amount, and most cars just give up and float away. At 2 feet (60 cm) of running water, vehicles are at risk of being swept away (even trucks and four-wheel drives). If flood waters start swirling around your vehicle, abandon it—and save your life.

AVOID THE UNKNOWN Beneath the water, the pavement might be ripped away, leaving a hole that could swallow your vehicle. The rule for driving through water is easy to remember: If you can't see the road surface or its line markings, take an alternate route.

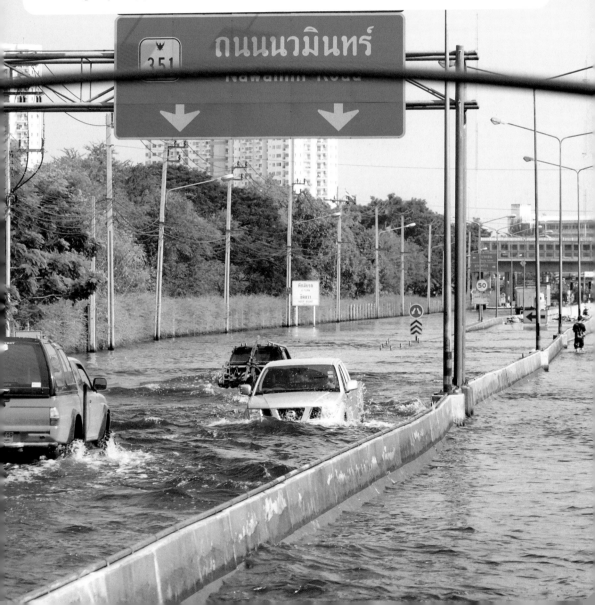

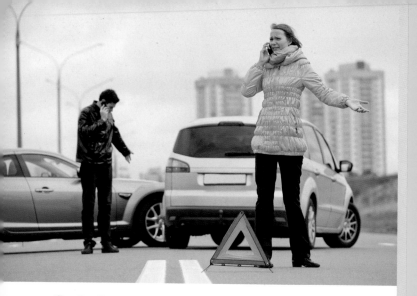

214 TEND TO A TRAFFIC ACCIDENT

Regardless of the specific details, getting into a car accident is unsettling. You're likely to feel overwhelmed or jittery, which can make doing the normal after-accident steps harder. Make a copy of these instructions, and store them with your insurance and registration to make everything as easy as possible for you.

☐ **GET OFF THE ROAD** Unless your vehicle is inoperable, or a police officer orders you to leave the vehicle in place, you should pull over to the roadside to a safe location. If that isn't possible, use your hazard lights if they're still functional.

☐ **CHECK FOR INJURY** Check to see if anyone has been hurt. If so, call for an ambulance and the police.

☐ **CALL THE POLICE** The police may not send an officer out to file a report for a minor accident, but you should still ask, and inform them if anyone involved appears agitated or hostile.

☐ **CALL A TOW TRUCK** Call for a tow truck for damaged vehicles.

☐ **GET INFO** Exchange information with others involved. Be sure to get:
- Driver's license information of everyone involved.
- Insurance policy information.
- Make, model, color, and license plate numbers of vehicles involved.
- Driver and passenger names and contact information.
- Contact info for any eyewitnesses.
- Name, badge number, and police department of any officers taking reports or investigating the accident.

☐ **TAKE PHOTOS** Take photographs of the incident.

☐ **FILE A CLAIM** Call your insurance company to file a claim.

215 SHOOT THE SCENE

One of the most important things that you can do at the scene of an accident is to take good pictures to document the incident. Doing so can help protect you from fraud and unfounded claims. Take as many photos as you can safely manage, from every angle.

First, get the big picture. Shoot the scene from far enough back that you can get everything in the shot, including skid marks, debris, and vehicles. You'll want to get multiple angles, so shoot from each side, as well as the front and rear.

Get some close-ups as well. Take pictures of all damage to all of the involved vehicles. Also, shoot each vehicle from all four sides (even if some sides show no damage) close enough that the entire vehicle fills the frame.

If there are any skid marks, get pictures of the vehicle that caused them, as well as the entirety of the skid marks. If you're not sure which vehicle caused the skid marks, take a picture of the skid marks with the accident in the background.

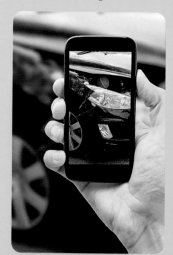

216 HELP A DOWNED RIDER

If you happen to be unlucky enough to be involved in an accident with a motorcyclist, or if you witness a downed rider there are a few things you should do while waiting for emergency responders to arrive.

If the motorcyclist is on the ground and injured, do not move them, and encourage them to remain still. Keep the rider's head and neck immobile and in a stable, neutral position until medical help arrives to take over care.

Have others help by directing traffic, laying out flares, or putting on their hazards and using their vehicles to protect the accident site.

If the victim is breathing normally, leave their helmet on. Remove the helmet only if the victim's airway is blocked or if they are not breathing.

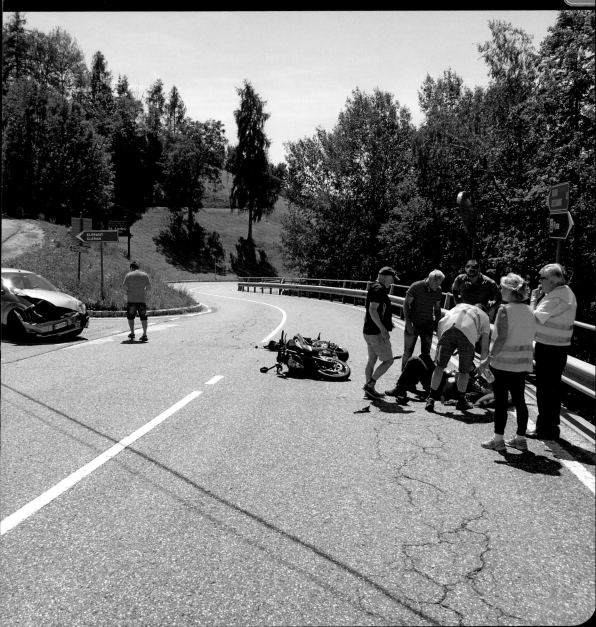

217 STAY SAFE IN TRANSIT

Situational awareness is the key to safety when taking public transportation of all sorts. Stay aware of your surroundings, and don't let yourself get lulled into zoning out and ignoring possible dangers. Here are some simple things you can do to increase your personal safety.

DON'T GO IT ALONE When waiting for a bus or train, stay in a central well-lit location with others nearby. After boarding, familiarize yourself with emergency buttons and exits, and ride near the driver or operator. Carry your cell phone at all times in case you need to call for help.

STAY ALERT Avoid falling asleep, and don't listen to music or talk on the phone. Likewise, avoid continuously using your phone, as it distracts you. Take a break from using it every minute to reevaluate your surroundings.

GUARD YOUR BELONGINGS Don't put your bags down on the seat next to you; keep them in your lap, under your arm, or between your feet. Avoid sitting right next to an exit door, as those seats are at higher risk for snatch-and-run thefts.

PROTECT YOURSELF Trust your instincts. Don't board or disembark if you're feeling unsafe. If someone bothers you or makes you uncomfortable, change seats, get off at the next stop, or change cars; notify the driver or operator if necessary. Consider carrying pepper spray or some other self-defense option.

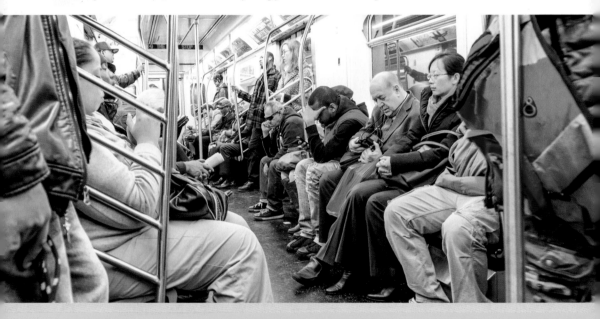

218 HANDLE HASSLE DISCREETLY

Is someone acting shady on the platform? Are people drunk on your subway car? Is a hustler hassling people by the ticket machines? If you're like most people, you won't want to risk confrontation but would welcome a way to report the issue quickly, easily, and discreetly. Luckily, smartphone apps are being released for various public transit systems that let you do just that. Check with your local public transit agency website or the app store for your smartphone to see if your area has released an app yet. Transit systems that have already implemented such a feature include Atlanta, Boston, Los Angeles, and the San Francisco Bay Area.

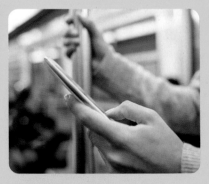

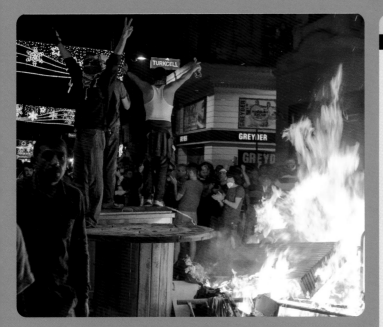

219 DON'T BE A BYSTANDER

The bystander effect describes the social and psychological phenomenon in which many bystanders observe an incident or are aware of a crime but no one acts to help the victim or even call for help. The more bystanders, the lower the chance anyone will do anything to help. Often this is because each person assumes that someone else is handling the problem. Sometimes they even manage to convince themselves that what's going on is no big deal, that the victim doesn't need any help. Everyone is potentially susceptible to this effect, but you can inoculate yourself to some extent.

BE PREPARED TO HELP By making the decision that you will step up to help if needed, you'll be primed to act if you should encounter such a circumstance (see item 38).

STAY AWARE Turn your awareness up to Orange, or even Red if the circumstance warrants it (see item 14). Carefully observe to ensure you have a clear and accurate understanding of what's happening. Do so discreetly and keep a 360-degree awareness to avoid being pulled into the incident.

CALL FOR HELP See if anyone is taking action to call for help. If not, do so yourself or ask someone to call for you. Take photos of participants if you can do so safely.

INTERVENE If you think you can make a difference, and you feel your safety isn't at risk, try yelling to stop the incident. If you're with a group of people, consider acting as a group to physically intervene.

ASSIST AFTERWARD Check on any victims to make sure they know help is on the way. Provide first aid if needed.

LIFE SAFETY APP
GPS

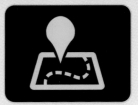

These days there are lots of options for GPS navigation. It's pretty common for people to have given up paper maps entirely in favor of their car's built-in GPS or a smartphone app. Regardless of whether you walk, drive, or use mass transit, consider upgrading your device to a GPS app that includes downloaded maps. While the basic mapping app the comes with your smart phone for free is perfectly fine for everyday use, after a natural disaster or other disruptive event you might lose your Internet or cell connection.

After an evacuation or while trying to avoid problem spots, you might find yourself traveling through or even stranded in an unfamiliar area with spotty data coverage and few resources. An app with downloaded maps will work even when your phone is totally offline, which can be a lifesaver. Even in a non-emergency situation you may find that your phone's basic mapping app doesn't work in rural or remote areas. When the signal drops just as you turn onto a winding dirt road in the middle of nowhere, it's nice to know that you have a backup.

SUGGESTED APPS
• *NAVIGON*
• *TomTom*
• *Sygic*
• *Google Maps* (in offline mode)

220 SURVIVE A SINKING SHIP

Whether you're commuting by ferry or on a cruise vacation, there's always the risk that your ship might sink. Luckily, large vessels don't sink quickly under most circumstances, giving you and the crew plenty of time to safely evacuate. But being prepared will improve your odds further. Follow these tactics to make abandoning ship as safe as possible.

ORIENT YOURSELF Get familiar with the layout of the ship, the closest lifeboats, and know where more than one exit is—your first choice may be underwater!

PACK A GO BAG Just as you already have done for your home or car, keep a small bag with essential items, including a whistle and a waterproof flashlight ready just in case you have to evacuate quickly.

LISTEN FOR A SIGN The international evacuation signal is seven short horn blasts followed by one long one. The crew may also use the intercom system to make any important announcements. If you can't hear instructions, head to an open deck level. Don't linger in the central or lower decks.

TAKE THE STAIRS Don't use an elevator unless there are no other options for evacuating safely. Electrical equipment may short out, or the ship's entire electrical system may fail, leaving you stranded inside an elevator at a time when rescue is unlikely.

LOOK BEFORE YOU LEAP If you're unable to board a lifeboat, look for a life preserver. Toss it into the water before you jump in after it. Look before you jump, as there may be people, lifeboats, debris, fire, or propellers in the water below that you could hit upon impact. Remember to jump feet first.

GET SOME DISTANCE Swim away from the ship as soon as you hit water. Falling debris and the vacuum effect created as the ship goes down can suck you under.

FIGHT BACK If in the water, kick and punch anything that brushes you from below. It might just be some debris from the ship, but why take the chance? It could be a shark, and striking it may be enough to deter an attack.

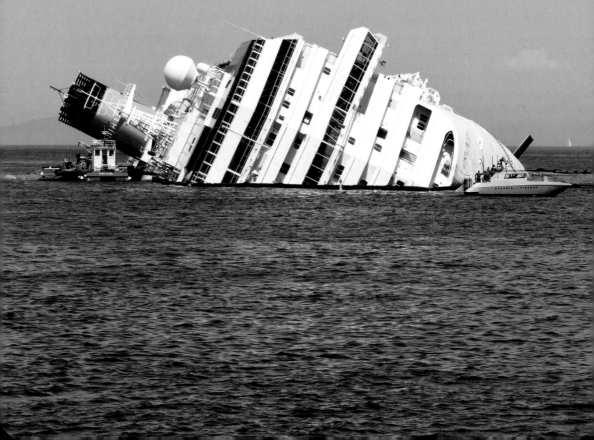

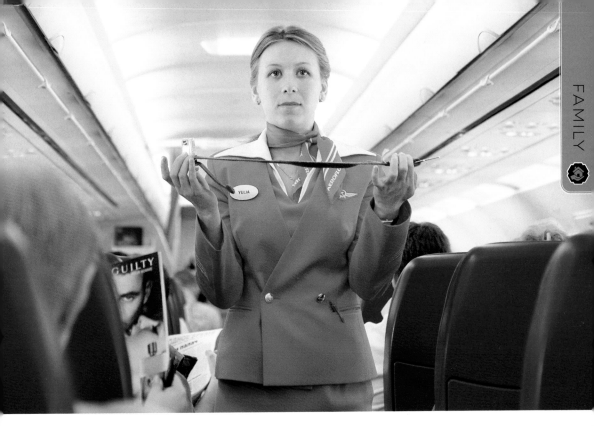

221 GET THROUGH A PLANE CRASH

If you're not the pilot, you may feel like there isn't much you can do to improve your chances of surviving a plane crash. However, statistics and crash investigations show that you can improve your chances by using these tactics.

DRESS RIGHT Whenever you fly, wear practical clothing, like a top with long sleeves, pants made of natural materials, and sturdy shoes. Proper clothing will help you to safely evacuate quickly and can protect you from sharp metal or flash burns, or if you have to run past burning jet fuel.

SIT TIGHT Sitting close to an exit gives you an advantage in an emergency evacuation. While every single crash is different, research has found that being within five rows of an exit gave passengers a higher chance of survival in some crashes. To improve your odds, sit in an aisle seat instead of next to the window. Crash statistics show that sitting in the back of a plane gives you higher odds of survival than in the front.

GET BRIEFED Every plane is different; listen to the safety briefing, read the safety card, and practice the brace position. During a crash you won't have time to review this material.

BUCKLE UP Keep your seat belt snugly buckled low on your hips when sitting in your seat. This will reduce kinetic injuries during impact as well as lower the risk of internal abdominal injuries.

KEEP ALERT Remain situationally aware during the first 3 minutes and the last 8 minutes of a flight, when there is the highest probability of a crash taking place. Keep your shoes on to give you an edge if you need to exit quickly.

INFLATE OUTSIDE Don't inflate your life vest until you're outside the cabin. If you do so while the plane is filling with water, you may get trapped instead of being able to swim out.

EXIT FAST In the event of fire, stay as low as you can and get out as quickly as possible. Your chances of survival are greatest if you can evacuate within 90 seconds.

GET SOME DISTANCE After evacuating from the plane, get as far away as reasonably possible in case of explosion. If the crash happens in a remote area, stay near the plane while awaiting rescue.

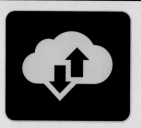

One key recommendation you should take away from this book is how crucial it is that you store all of your important documents safely. You should keep original physical copies of things like birth certificates, social security cards, bank documents, and other key items in a secure location, and a full set of duplicate photocopies in a second location, in case the first is destroyed or inaccessible in an emergency.

Given how easy it is to scan documents into PDF files these days, consider installing a cloud storage app on your smartphone so that you'll have easy access to all of your important files even if you're away from home or don't have access to the backup copies. If you're concerned about cloud security, you can use two-factor authentication to help keep your data more secure than it would be with just a password. There are many different options available, but three popular ones with free storage options are Dropbox, Google Drive, and Box.

SUGGESTED APPS
• *Dropbox*
• *Google Drive*
• *Box*

222 BUCKET UP

If the water and power go out while you're sheltering in place, that means your toilet won't work. If you don't have an outhouse, you'll need a sanitary way to easily manage human waste.

Buy thick plastic trash bags, a small bag of kitty litter, some toilet paper, duct tape, a permanent marker, disposable gloves, hand sanitizer, and a 5-gallon (19-liter) painter's bucket. (Also, you can optionally buy a special toilet seat from disaster supply stores that fits on the bucket.) Place all of the supplies inside the bucket except one of the plastic bags. Seal the bucket and place it into the plastic bag to keep moisture out, and keep it in storage.

When you need to use the bucket, double-bag the inside, and sprinkle kitty litter generously after each use. When the bucket is about half full, seal the inner bag with a knot, then tie the outer bag with another knot, then finally seal the knot with duct tape and write "Human Waste" on the duct tape with the marker. Place bags someplace out of the way, preferably out of direct sunlight. Check local regulations on how to properly dispose of waste after services are restored.

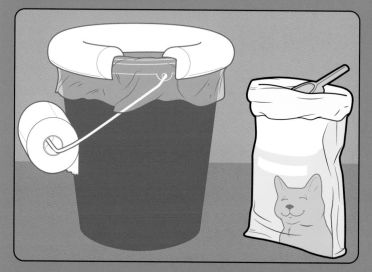

223 ADDRESS BOOK IT

Having copies of your family disaster and communication plans on your smartphone can be useful when you need to get out of town quickly or have to contact your out-of-town emergency family contact pronto. The only thing is, you don't want to have to spend valuable time scrolling for that information in different places. Program all information in your phone's address book with an entry name like "Emergency Family Contact" or "Evacuation Destination" to make finding all the relevant information as fast and easy as possible. Include map links, notes, and other important data in the entry as well and you'll be good to go.

224 MAKE A DATE TO PREPARE

If you find the idea of comprehensive disaster preparedness too overwhelming or time-consuming, an easy way to make it manageable is to space the different tasks throughout the year so that everything gets done and checked annually. On the first of each month, check this handy calendar and schedule the month's activities with your family.

MONTH	CATEGORY	KEY TASK	REVIEW
JANUARY	COMMUNICATION PLAN	Discuss and create plans with your household	Review plans with everyone in the household
FEBRUARY	WATER SUPPLY	Review normal water supply; create a five-to-seven-day disaster supply	Replace water supply as needed
MARCH	FOOD SUPPLY	Review pantry; establish a five-to-seven-day disaster food supply	Replace food supply as needed
APRIL	EVACUATION ROUTES	Determine two escape routes from your house and the region	Review plans with everyone in the household
MAY	FIRST AID KIT	Gather necessary supplies	Review kit; replace used supplies; add other supplies if needed
JUNE	DOCUMENTS AND KEYS	Make copies of important documents and keys	Review keys and documents; update or replace if needed
JULY	EQUIPMENT AND TOOLS	Check current setup; purchase any needed items to complete the kit	Replace any missing items
AUGUST	SANITATION AND HYGIENE	Gather supplies in a large waterproof container	Replace any expired items
SEPTEMBER	MEDICINE KIT	Review everyone's prescription needs; create a disaster backup supply	Rotate the backup supply before medications expire
OCTOBER	CLOTHING AND BEDDING	Pack clothing (options for warm, wet, and cold weather) and bedding for each person	Ensure clothes still fit; inspect for damage and wash items if needed
NOVEMBER	HOME HAZARDS	Identify hazards in and outside home; mitigate if possible	Review existing hazards; search for new ones
DECEMBER	PET EMERGENCY SUPPLIES	Establish a five-to-seven-day food supply	Replace supplies and food as needed

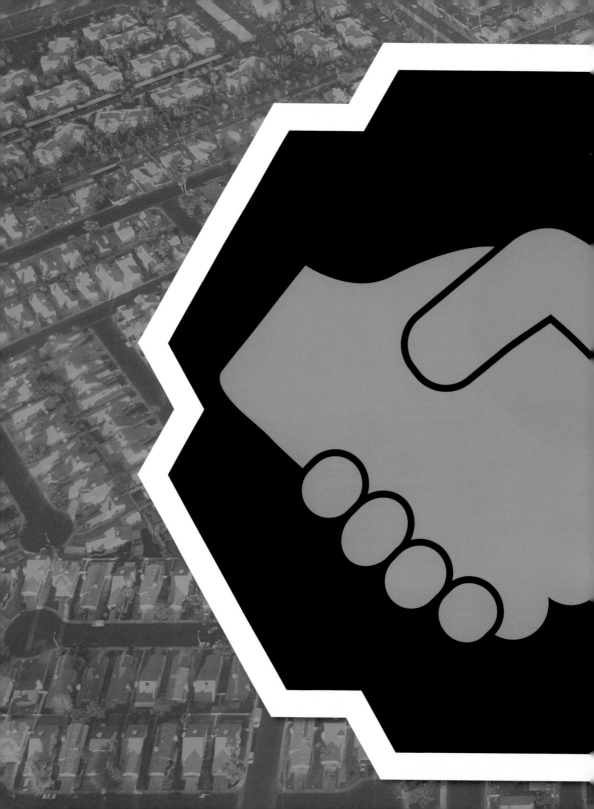

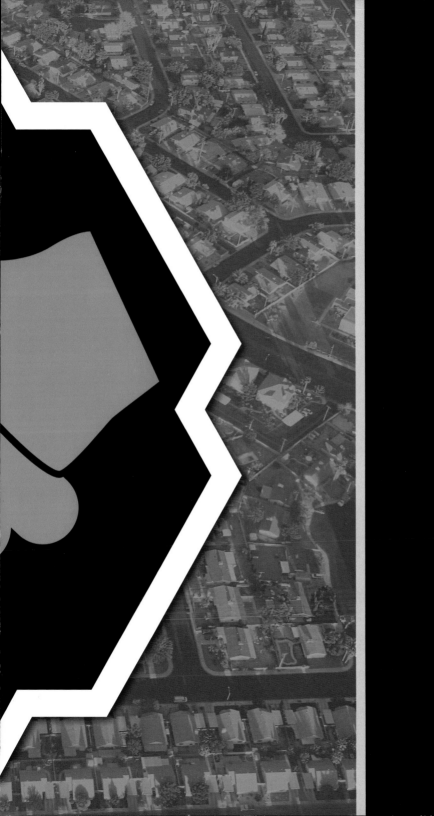

COMMUNITY

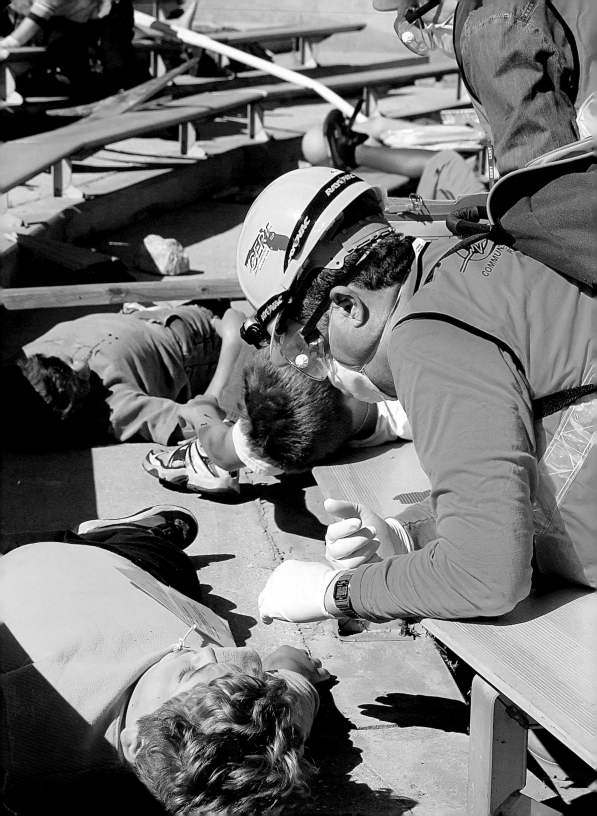

SOMETIMES THE ONLY WAY TO LEARN HOW YOU'LL MANAGE IN A CRISIS IS ACTUALLY TO BE IN ONE.

Very early one morning several decades ago, when I was first learning how to drive my 4X4, we ended up stuck axel-deep in mud in the middle of nowhere in a high desert. We decided that since we were beyond the range of cell phones or two-way radio we would send one person to hike back to the nearest town, quite a distance away, while the rest of us attempted to dig the truck out. We had no luck digging out the truck—the tools we had weren't sufficient. So we were very grateful when, later in the afternoon, a couple of vehicles from the town showed up to help pull us out. Having and executing a plan B significantly shortened the time we were stranded and gave me a valuable lesson in just how good my resources were. Future expeditions were better equipped and planned and because of that I've never needed to dig myself out since.

Natural disasters and large-scale regional events will have a significant impact on your local community, especially on emergency resources. If you're not prepared, you'll be one of the many thousands clamoring for food, water, shelter, and supplies. It's a situation you never want to be in, but if you take advantage of the local emergency management information about hazards in your area and have prepared a five-to-seven-day kit you'll be able to handle the challenge. Wondering about natural disasters? This section covers the gamut, from earthquakes and volcanoes, to hurricanes and tornados. Should you stay or should you go? Learn about survival priorities, evacuation, shelter-in-place, as well as additional strategies for food and water. What about other risks? RRead about how to become better prepared for chemical spills, solar flares, and pandemics. Lastly, this section prepares you to take the next step; to become a resilient survivor of whatever Mother Nature or man-made disaster affects your region.

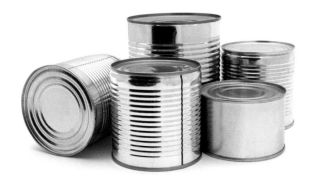

225 AVOID A WORLD OF TROUBLE

This map shows some of the most commonly occurring natural disasters and where you're likely to find them.

VOLCANOES Activity occurs largely around the "Ring of Fire," the Pacific region that includes Hawaii and Japan. A second active area extends from Java all the way through the Himalayas and the Mediterranean.

EARTHQUAKES Most commonly occurring along the edge of the earth's tectonic plates, quakes can also be caused by volcanic activity, landslides, mining, fracking, and drilling.

HURRICANES Also known as cyclones or typhoons, these tropical storms can have a wide range, as they are propelled north and south by massively powerful winds.

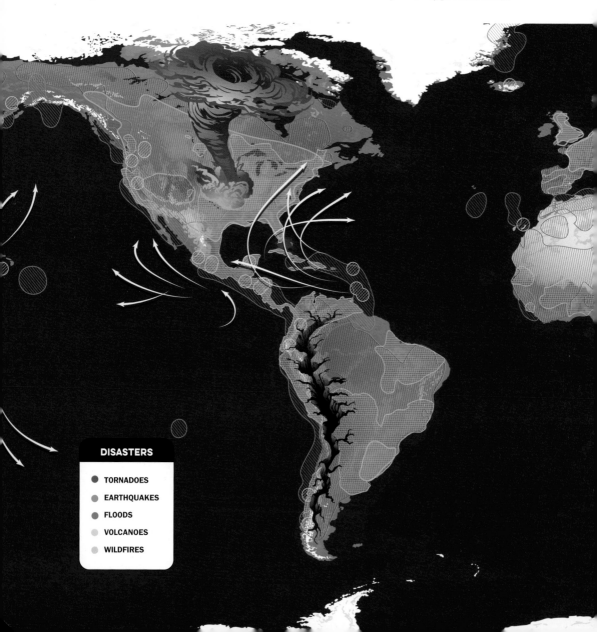

DISASTERS

- TORNADOES
- EARTHQUAKES
- FLOODS
- VOLCANOES
- WILDFIRES

FLOODS While flooding can be caused by a number of factors, including dams failing or dikes being breached, in the natural world, flooding follows seasonal snowmelt and storms, and can occur anywhere rain falls heavily.

WILDFIRES Not only triggered by lightning or human error, wildfires are becoming more common around the world as the climate changes and more frequent periods of drought and dry seasons increase fire risk.

TORNADOES Tornadoes happen when the right confluence of thunderstorms and complex air patterns come together. They devastate the central and southern United States and are common in Europe and Australia as well.

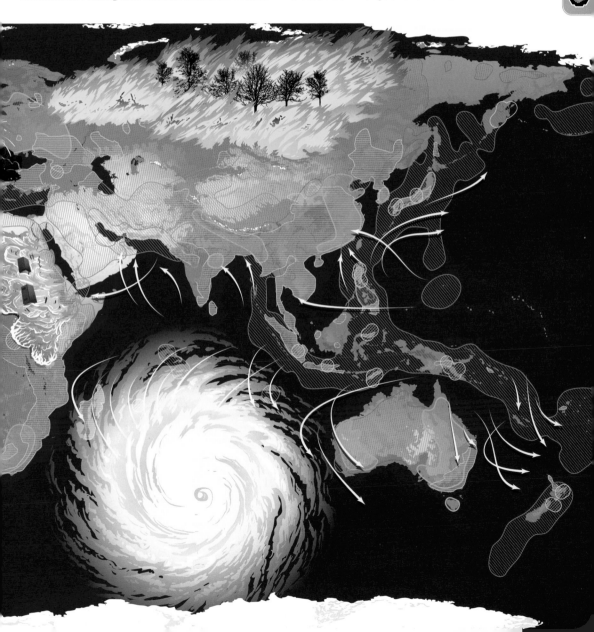

226 CHART YOUR PRIORITIES

Knowing how to prioritize for a given disaster is important so that you don't end up focusing on the wrong thing and wasting what time you may have to prepare for your own safety. Start with the first priority and work your way down the list. Circumstances may change quickly; be prepared to adapt to changing conditions.

DISASTER	1	2	3
TSUNAMI	If imminent, get to high ground immediately.	Check Internet, weather radio, or broadcast media for news that affects your area.	Prepare to evacuate; gather supplies and go bags.
EARTHQUAKE	Get to a safe place: Drop, cover, and hold on!	Stay there until it's safe, or leave if it's too dangerous to stay.	Shut off utilities after the quake.
FLOODING		Prepare to evacuate; gather supplies and go bags.	Learn the safe evacuation route, if needed.
TORNADO		Seek cover in a shelter or an interior windowless room.	Await the all-clear signal via siren, Internet, or news.
HURRICANE	Check Internet, weather radio, or broadcast media for news in your area.	If time allows, board up windows; sandbag and secure your home.	Gather supplies and go bags.
VOLCANO		Decide whether to shelter in place or evacuate.	Gather supplies and go bags.
PANDEMIC		Avoid close contact with people who are sick.	Wear medical gloves, goggles, and N95 masks when in public.
WILDFIRES		Fill up the gas tank in the vehicle intended for evacuation.	Gather supplies and go bags.
POWER FAILURE		Activate solar chargers or prepare portable emergency generators.	Gather supplies and go bags.
HAZARDOUS MATERIALS/ NUCLEAR INCIDENT		Decide to either shelter in place or evacuate.	Seal windows, doors, and vents with plastic and duct tape.

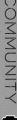

4	5
Secure your home; move valuable items to the highest floor.	Shut off utilities.
Seek shelter if your home is no longer safe.	Inventory supplies.
Secure and sandbag your home.	Consider proactively evacuating.
Assess if your area is still at risk.	Evacuate to another shelter if yours is no longer sound.
Decide whether to shelter in place or evacuate.	If evacuating, shut off utilities before leaving.
Wear goggles and dust masks to protect your eyes and airway.	Seal doors, windows, and ducts against ash; turn off fans and air conditioners.
Gather extra food and medical supplies in case of a long quarantine.	Consider evacuating to an unaffected area if supplies are low.
Shut off gas main; turn off propane tanks.	Consider proactively evacuating.
Inventory supplies.	Ration battery-powered devices to maximize operational life.
Gather supplies and go bags.	Be ready to cut off and discard any clothes that may be contaminated; have spare clothing handy.

227 TAKE ONLY WHAT YOU CAN

The worst disasters you'll encounter will force you to make some difficult decisions about your home, your belongings, and your loved ones.

When facing imminent evacuation along with the possibility of losing your home, you'll have to decide which personal items, family heirlooms, and pictures you want to take with you. If you haven't thought about this in advance, when disaster strikes, you may lose valuable time trying to decide and gather these things, risking your own safety in the process. Ask yourself, if I could only take one thing with me, what would it be? In some circumstances, you'll have just enough time to evacuate with your go bag and not much else.

While you will likely have more time, it's useful to plan ahead to recognize what you can reasonably take with you, given time and space constraints.

If you have a written family plan, consider adding a checklist of the items that each family member feels is important to bring along so that if they happen to be away from home, and time allows, someone else can gather those sentimental items well in advance.

Worst yet, if you have a lot of pets, especially larger ones that don't fit easily into your car, you may be forced to leave one or more behind. Discuss this with your family members in advance so if the worst does happen, this difficult topic won't create more conflict or delay a safe evacuation. If you know beforehand that certain pets or animals can't come along, make sure you have a plan and the necessary supplies to responsibly leave them behind. It isn't ideal, but you may have no choice, and disasters often necessitate difficult decisions.

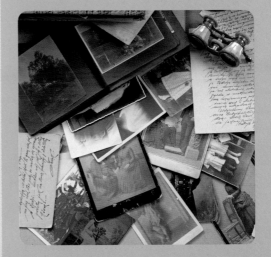

228 DECIDE TO STAY (OR GO)

The decision whether to shelter in place or evacuate could be the toughest and most important decision you make in the time before, during, or after a disaster. While certain types of disasters require evacuation, some situations are best ridden out in a secure, well-provisioned home or place of business. That said, the circumstances may dictate that evacuation really will be the best (or only) choice. Here is a simple model to help you decide if it's time for you to dig in for the long haul, or if you should haul out of there instead.

IF	
Authorities announce that your area should evacuate	Authorities announce that you should shelter in place
OR	
The situation is worsening and you decide that travel is safer than staying	The situation is not safe enough to travel through
AND	
You have an evacuation plan	You don't have a means to leave the area, or traffic won't allow you to leave
AND	
You have the necessary gear and supplies	You have a prepared disaster kit of gear and supplies
OR	
You are meeting up with others who are better prepared and equipped	You have nowhere else to go
THEN	
EVACUATE	SHELTER IN PLACE

229 EVACUATE EARLY

A number of disaster types can have hours—and on some occasions, days—of notice prior to impacting your area. Some examples include hurricanes, floods, wildfires, winter storms, tsunamis, and even volcanic eruptions. While it's tempting to wait and see if you really need to evacuate, the possible consequence of waiting is being trapped in the disaster area, which may place you and your family at risk. Additionally, the longer you wait to evacuate, the more snarled traffic will be on the designated evacuation routes. Leaving early allows you to stay ahead of the problem in some cases, which can make the experience of evacuating less stressful for some.

Depending on the reason for evacuating, you should consider turning off your gas, electricity, and water before leaving. If you decide to keep your electricity running, switch off the breakers for any circuits that aren't powering something critical, such as the freezer and refrigerator.

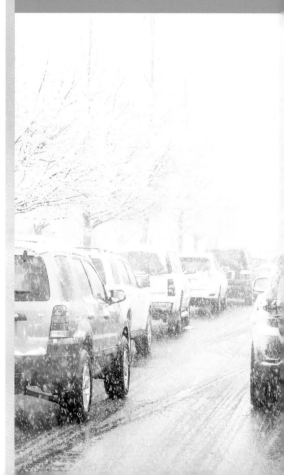

230 SIGNAL FOR HELP

If you shelter in place, or if you get stranded and need to signal for help, knowing some of the international signals recognized by pilots will allow you to call for help even if you don't carry a personal locator beacon (PLB) or a satellite phone (see item 163). These signals are passive and will allow any search aircraft to understand your needs even if you're not actively signaling for help. Other forms of signaling, such as smoke, flares, and fires, are also effective but may not be suitable or safe for urban use, such as on a rooftop. Consider keeping several cans of spray paint to mark the ground or roof. If you must improvise, you can also use things such as fabric, branches, wood, debris, or any other material that will contrast sharply with the ground. Alternatively, you can dig the patterns into the ground. Make the symbols as large as you can using the materials available, ideally building the symbols to about 20 feet (6m) in height.

X	Require medical assistance
V	Require assistance
F	Require food and water
L	Require fuel and oil
W	Require repair
LL	All is well
→	Proceeding in this direction
▲	Believe safe to land here
SOS	General distress signal

231 WAVE FOR HELP

If you are in visual range of an aircraft and you wish to signal to them using your arms, here are the two main signals you need to know.

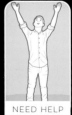
NEED HELP

ALL OKAY

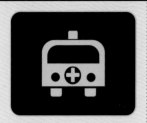

232 KNOW YOUR WEATHER ALERTS

The National Weather Service has developed a multi-tier system to notify the public of threatening weather conditions, and knowing the difference between these terms can help you understand the information and make better decisions about the relative risk you might be exposed to.

OUTLOOK A Hazardous Weather Outlook is issued daily to indicate that a hazardous weather event may occur in the next several days. The outlook will usually consist of information about the specific threat (such as severe thunderstorms, flooding, winter weather, or extremes of heat or cold) that may develop over the next week, with an emphasis on the following 24 hours of the outlook. It provides advance notice for those needing considerable lead time to prepare for the event. Outlooks are an excellent opportunity to review and update your disaster supplies.

WATCH A watch is used when the risk of a hazardous weather event has increased significantly, but its occurrence, location, or timing is still not certain. Issuing a watch means that hazardous weather is possible. Watches are a good time for you to review your communication, shelter-in-place, and evacuation plans. Monitor weather updates, especially if planning travel or outdoor activities.

ADVISORY An advisory is issued when a hazardous weather event is occurring, imminent, or likely. Advisories are for less serious conditions than warnings. However, they may cause significant inconvenience and, if caution is not exercised, could lead to injuries or property damage.

WARNING A warning is issued when a hazardous weather event is occurring, imminent, or likely. A warning means weather conditions pose a threat to life or property; activating your emergency action plan may be necessary.

STATEMENT A statement is either issued as a follow-up message that may update, extend, or cancel a previous message or a notification of significant weather for which no type of advisory, watch, or warning exists.

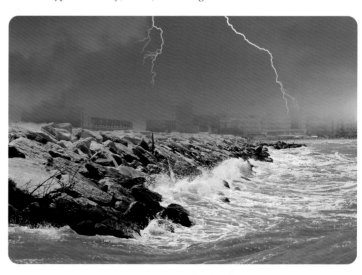

233 CATEGORIZE WEATHER ALERTS

The National Weather Service divides severe weather alerts into a different categories of hazardous weather and hydrologic events.

SEVERE LOCAL STORMS Short-fused, small-scale hazardous weather or any events produced by thunderstorms, including large hail, damaging winds, tornadoes, and flash floods.

WINTER STORMS Weather hazards associated with frozen precipitation (freezing rain, sleet, snow) or the combined effects of precipitation and strong winds.

FIRE WEATHER Weather conditions leading to an increased risk of wildfires.

FLOODING Hazardous hydrologic events resulting in flooding of land areas not normally covered by water, often caused by excessive rainfall.

COASTAL OR LAKESHORE HAZARDS Hydrological hazards in areas near ocean and lake waters including high surf and coastal or lakeshore flooding, as well as rip currents.

MARINE HAZARDS Hazardous events that may affect boats and ships along large bodies of water, such as rough seas and freezing spray.

OTHER HAZARDS Examples include extreme heat or cold, dense fog, high winds, and river or lakeshore flooding.

234 HEED WARNING FLAGS

If you're near or on the water, it's good to know what these flags mean, since they are used to visually communicate weather conditions.

WARNING FLAG	CATEGORY	DESCRIPTION	WIND KNOTS	WIND MPH	WIND KPH	WAVE HEIGHT FT (M)
	SMALL CRAFT ADVISORY	Strong Breeze	22–27	25–31	40–50	9.9 (3)
		High Wind	28–33	32–38	51–61	13 (4)
	GALE WARNING	Gale	34–40	39–46	62–74	18 (5.5)
		Severe Gale	41–47	47–54	75–87	23 (7)
	STORM WARNING	Storm	48–55	55–63	88–100	30 (9)
		Violent Storm	56–63	64–72	101–116	38 (11.5)
	HURRICANE WARNING	Hurricane	64+	73+	117+	46 (14)

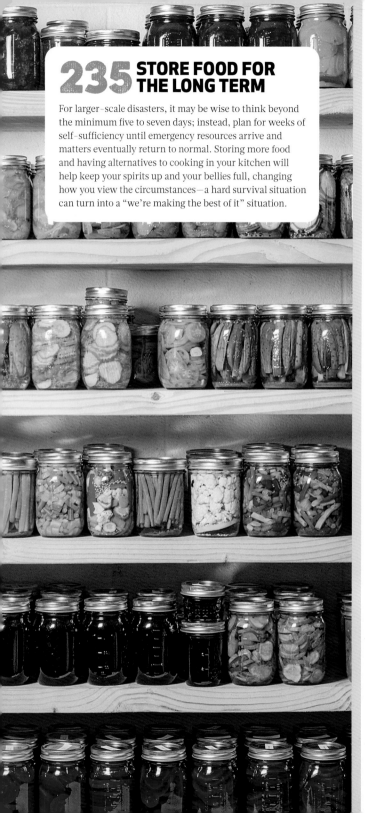

235 STORE FOOD FOR THE LONG TERM

For larger-scale disasters, it may be wise to think beyond the minimum five to seven days; instead, plan for weeks of self-sufficiency until emergency resources arrive and matters eventually return to normal. Storing more food and having alternatives to cooking in your kitchen will help keep your spirits up and your bellies full, changing how you view the circumstances—a hard survival situation can turn into a "we're making the best of it" situation.

236 PACK IT UP RIGHT

For long-term storage of dry goods, consider using containers made of PETE (polyethylene terephthalate) plastic. You can find plenty of standard containers made with PETE (listed under the recycling symbol on the label), but buy fresh ones; don't reuse old food or drink containers. Some plastic is just too flimsy or susceptible to moisture, oxygen, and pests, but PETE, when used in combination with oxygen-absorbing packets, will do the job. You should only use this kind of packaging for dry goods—moist foods must be handled differently to avoid the risk of botulism. Containers should be no bigger than 1 gallon (4 liters) for optimal effectiveness.

STEP 1 Test your container's seal by closing it tightly, placing it under water, and pressing on the lid or cap. If any bubbles escape, the seal is faulty, and you shouldn't use it for long-term storage.

STEP 2 Place an oxygen absorber (a packet of iron powder that helps keep food fresh; you can purchase these at home-storage stores or online) in the container.

STEP 3 Fill your container with dry goods (wheat, corn, dry beans, etc).

STEP 4 Wipe the bottle's top sealing edge clean with a dry cloth, and then press the lid on tightly.

STEP 5 Store the sealed container in a cool, dry location away from direct light. If you use a container's contents, add a new oxygen absorber when you refill it.

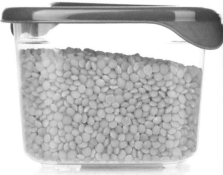

237 COOK IN A DISASTER

During a large-scale disaster you may have to survive for a while without electricity or gas to cook with in your kitchen. If you do still have electricity, a microwave can provide you an option for cooking. If you have neither gas nor electricity, you need alternatives. In an urban area you may not be able to light a fire outside, and your nearby parks with grills and fire pits might already be taken over by others.

If your house has a fireplace, you can use it to cook if you have a way to hold the pots and pans over the fire. If you have a backyard grill, store extra fuel for use in a disaster. Consider also adding a small hibachi to your disaster supplies. Place it on bricks or baking sheets to protect the surface below the grill.

Camping stoves come in various sizes and designs, and they operate on a variety of fuel types, some of which may even be safe to use indoors (check before you buy). If you have one for camping that's also safe to be used indoors, you'll be set when disaster strikes. Sterno fuel is also safe to use indoors, but it won't provide as much heat as other stove options. You can warm foods, but boiling water might be a challenge.

There are also wood-burning backpack stoves designed to effectively burn twigs and branches, making fuel supply less of an issue. Solar stoves can be made from household items if you opt not to buy a commercial model; they don't require fuel per se, but they won't work at night or when it's overcast. Avoid solid-fuel stoves due to the toxic nature of the fuel pellets and the gases they release upon being burned.

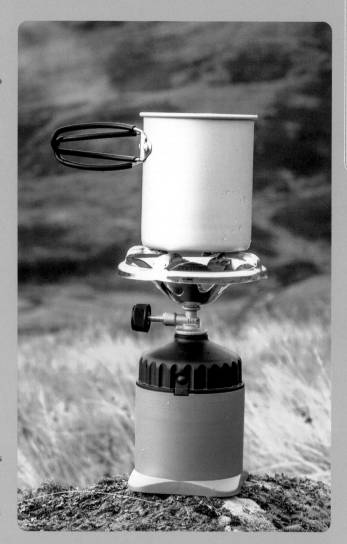

238 KEEP YOUR STASH FRESH

A basic rule of any food pantry is "first in, first out." What that means is, keep track of the expiration dates on items, and use them shortly before that date. For example, those canned goods that are good for another year? After eleven months, replace them and use them to make dinner. You should never have to throw anything away; just keep using the ingredients and replace them as needed. That way, if or when disaster does strike, your food won't be spoiled, and you won't go hungry.

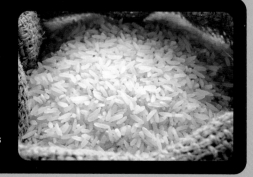

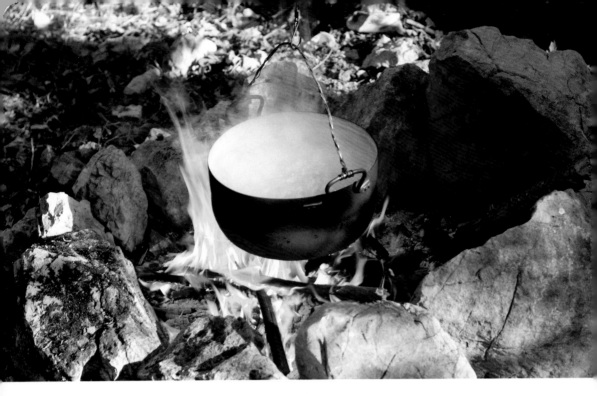

239 PURIFY WATER

If you have used up all of your stored water and there are no other reliable clean-water sources, it may become necessary to treat any unknown water source to make it potable. Treat all water, no matter what you plan on using it for. Besides potentially having a bad odor and taste, contaminated water can contain microorganisms as well as other contaminants.

There are several ways to treat water, but none of them are perfect, so if time and resources allow, the best practice is to combine methods. Before treating, filter debris and particulates by using cheesecloth, coffee filters, or available clean cloth.

USE ULTRAVIOLET The ultraviolet (UV) light water treatment is fast and easy, and you can use a special UV light device (see item 244) or sunlight. To treat up to 33 ounces (1 liter) at a time, just stir the device for 90 seconds in the water and it's ready for you to drink.

BOIL IT This is the safest method of treating water, achieved by simply bringing water to a rolling boil for 5 minutes. The water will taste better if you aerate it by pouring the water back and forth between two clean containers.

TRY CHLORINE Use only regular household liquid bleach containing 5.25 to 6.0 percent sodium hypochlorite. Do not use bleach that is scented, color safe, or has added cleansers. Use a newly opened or unopened bottle, as the potency of bleach diminishes with time. Add 8 drops of bleach for each gallon (4 liters) of water, stir, and let stand for 30 minutes. The water should have a slight bleach odor. If not, repeat the dosage and let stand another 15 minutes. If it still does not smell of chlorine, discard it and find another source of water.

DISTILL IT Distillation has the advantage of removing other contaminants besides microbes but unfortunately is also the most complicated method of treating water unless you own a distiller unit (which may not work if power is unavailable).

METHOD	KILLS MICROBES	REMOVES OTHER CONTAMINANTS*
UV LIGHT		No
BOILING	Yes	No
CHLORINATION	Yes	
DISTILLATION		Yes

* HEAVY METALS, SALTS, AND OTHER CHEMICALS

240 TRY SOLAR DISINFECTION

If you have a clear glass or plastic bottle, some water, and a sunny day, you can harness the power of the sun's light to make your water much safer to drink. Largely advocated for developing countries, solar water disinfection is also useful in any post–disaster circumstance anywhere in the world, although it's best applied in equatorial countries that can provide abundant strong sunlight.

The most common solar disinfection technique is to expose a clear plastic bottle full of questionable water to the sun for a minimum of one full day. The sun's natural UV light kills or damages almost all biological contaminants in the water. This method is easy to do, it's essentially free, and it offers good (but not complete) bacterial and viral disinfection.

Use only clear bottles that are 66 ounces (2 liters) or smaller in size for effective treatment. The water must be clear, so filter it first if necessary. Set the water bottle out in direct sunlight for an entire day, or leave it out for two days if the weather is overcast.

There are some challenges, though: This method is not effective in rainy weather. It offers no residual disinfection and is not as effective against bacterial spores and cyst stages of some parasites. It's not 100 percent effective, but it's better than taking your chances with untreated water.

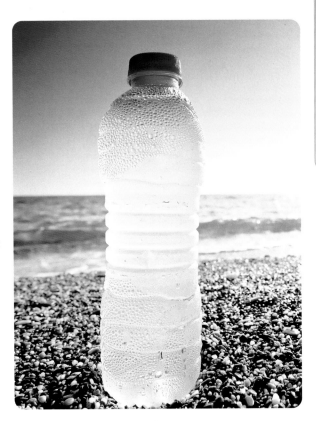

241 DISTILL WATER PROPERLY

Distillation is simple in principle, involving boiling water and then collecting the vapor that condenses. If you lack special lab equipment or a commercial distiller, you can improvise using a large pot, some paracord, and a mug.

STEP 1 Fill the pot halfway with water.

STEP 2 Tie the cup to the handle on the pot's lid so that the cup will hang right side up while the lid is upside down. Check to be sure that, when you lower the lid, the cup is not dangling into the water. If possible, add some ice to the inverted lid to speed up condensation below.

STEP 3 Boil the water for 20 minutes.

STEP 4 Carefully lift the lid. The water that has dripped from the lid into the cup is distilled and safe to drink.

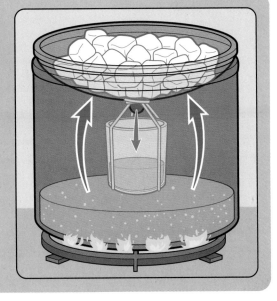

242 USE A STERIPEN

As we've already discussed, the standard methods for purifying water are safe, but they're rarely portable, fast, or battery powered. This is especially true if you're on the move and can't bring liquid bleach or a stove, or don't have the time to treat water with sunlight. The challenge of safe drinking water leaves you with few options if you want something for when you're on the move. The SteriPEN, however, is the answer. SteriPEN products are compact UV light generators that purify water by destroying more than 99.9 percent of bacteria, viruses, and even protozoan cysts such as giardia and cryptosporidia. The type recommended for disaster use is powered by AA batteries, since those are more common than the more expensive CR123 batteries and easier than the rechargeable options. With alkaline batteries it will treat about 13 gallons (50 liters), and with lithium AA batteries it can treat up to 39 gallons (150 liters). SteriPENs can treat up to a quarter of a gallon (1 liter) at a time. Just filter the water to remove particulate matter and debris, then submerge and stir for approximately 90 seconds until the SteriPEN display advises that the treatment is complete. Your water is now safe to drink.

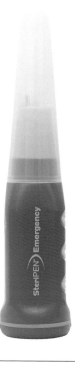

243 MAKE NORMAL SALINE

Normal saline can be used as a sterile rinse, disinfectant, and mouthwash. It should be made using non-iodized salt purchased from the grocery store; rock salt or sea salt are not recommended for this purpose. If available, use distilled or purified water instead of tap water. Since the homemade saline solution will only be effective for about a day, it's best to only make enough needed for immediate use.

STEP 1 If you plan on pouring the solution into a container, sterilize it by boiling tap water and placing the container and the lid in the water for 15 minutes.

STEP 2 Turn off the heat and let it sit, 15-30 minutes until the water has cooled.

STEP 3 Remove the container without touching the inside of the container, lid, or lip.

STEP 4: METRIC Boil 1 liter of distilled or purified water and add 9 grams of salt.

STEP 4: IMPERIAL Add ½ teaspoon of salt per cup of distilled or purified water.

STEP 5 Allow to boil for 15 minutes with the lid on and then let cool.

STEP 6 Label the outside of the container with the date and discard after a day.

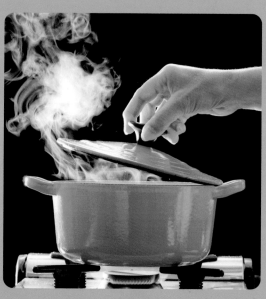

244 DISINFECT WITH BLEACH

During a longer-duration disaster or in a pandemic, you'll have limited resources to disinfect reusable supplies and equipment. One way to disinfect is to create a 1:100 bleach solution from chlorine with a base strength of 5 percent. If you don't have the means to easily measure the right amount of bleach, you can do so using a cup measure and two buckets.

STEP 1 Using a Sharpie, mark one bucket 1:10 and the other 1:100 in large block numbers.

STEP 2 Add 9 cups (2 liters) of water to the 1:10 bucket.

STEP 3 Carefully add 1 cup (200 mL) bleach to the water. You've now created a 1:10 bleach solution. Like regular bleach, 1:10 bleach is caustic and should be stored in a safe place with a lid over it.

STEP 4 In the 1:100 bucket, add 9 cups (2 liters) of water and then pour 1 cup (200 mL) of the 1:10 bleach solution to create a solution of 1:100.

You can now use this solution to disinfect a variety of things. Both solutions must be prepared daily, as they lose their strength after 24 hours. If the chlorine smell is not detectable, discard the solution as expired.

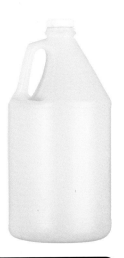

DISINFECT	BLEACH SOLUTION	SOAK TIME	NOTES
GLOVES	1:100	1 minute	Rinse in water afterward.
THERMOMETERS		10 minutes	Let air dry.
STETHOSCOPES		—	Wipe with solution-soaked cloth.
UTENSILS		—	Wash in soap and water, rinse in solution, then air dry.
INFECTIOUS WASTE SPILL		15 minutes	Remove with a cloth soaked in 1:100, then wash with soap and water afterward.
HARD SURFACES (tables, sinks, walls, floor)		—	Mop first with soap and water, then use the bleach solution.
LAUNDRY		30 minutes	After soaking in bleach, soak items in soapy water overnight.
MAJOR INFECTIOUS WASTE SPILL	1:10	15 minutes	Use a higher concentration if a known pandemic pathogen is suspected.

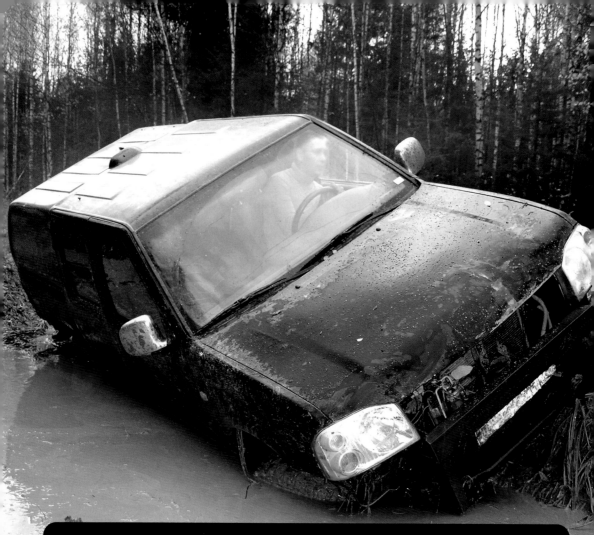

245 GET OUT OF THE MUD

During and after flooding, silt and mud make driving difficult, and you risk getting bogged down in mud. Likely, your vehicle will sink to the axles and refuse to move. Even if you're prepared, it will take time and effort to free your vehicle. Here's how to do get moving again.

GET OFF THE GAS Spinning your tires will only end up digging deeper ruts and tossing around the remaining solid ground under the wheels.

GO BACK AND FORTH Switch between reverse and first gear to rock the vehicle; the wheels may pick up enough traction to get you out. Try it a few times.

DIG A PATH Using whatever tools you have on hand, hollow out a hole in the mud in front of each tire. Give each hole a slightly upward slope, then drive forward very gently and, with any luck, up the incline.

MAKE TRACTION Search your vehicle and the surrounding environment for items such as branches, gravel, blankets, or even your floor mats, and lay them immediately ahead of the wheels. Then gently drive over these objects onto firmer ground.

KEEP MOVING Once free, don't stop until you're back on firm ground.

246 CROSS FAST-MOVING WATER

Sometimes you may not be able to wait around for someone to build a safe water crossing. Fording swift-moving water can be dangerous, but if you apply some basic triangular geometry, it can help you cross safely. If you are braving the current and you are backed up by two friends onshore—with a sturdy loop of rope twice the width of the body of water connecting all three of you—the two on land will be able to help you, even if you lose your footing. Once you reach the far bank, the second can cross, using the rope stretched between the banks as a safety line. When the last person is ready to cross, they enter the water and can be pulled across by the two on the far shore holding the rope.

Other tips for safety: Face upstream while you cross. Leave your shoes on to protect your feet and give you better grip. Shuffle your feet along the bottom, and avoid lifting your feet. If the conditions are not favorable at one site, look for a better spot to cross.

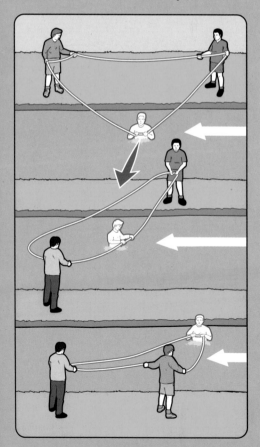

247 ASSESS YOUR HOME AFTER A FLOOD

When the all-clear sounds, you'll need to return home and assess the damage. But even after the waters recede, you may still be in danger. Follow these basic guidelines to stay safe.

BE SURE OF STABILITY If doors are stuck in their frames, or if your foundation or roof looks damaged, you should wait for an inspector to check out your home's stability before you go back inside.

AIR IT OUT If it appears safe to enter, open doors and windows to air out your home. Assist in drying the interior by using fans and dehumidifiers to help remove excess moisture.

CHECK FOR GAS LEAKS If there is a strong smell of natural gas or if you hear a hissing sound, immediately exit, opening any doors and windows as you leave to air out the house. Turn off the gas main and then remain outside. Have either the fire department or gas utility check your home before reentering.

POWER ON WITH CARE If the floor is wet, turn off the power at the main circuit breaker or fuse box with a nonconductive item, such as a broom handle or a rolled-up rubber floormat. Have an electrician inspect appliances or anything electrical or motorized that got wet prior to turning them back on.

SPOT SAGGING Check the ceiling and floor for any signs of sagging. Water may be trapped in the ceiling, or floors may be unsafe to walk on.

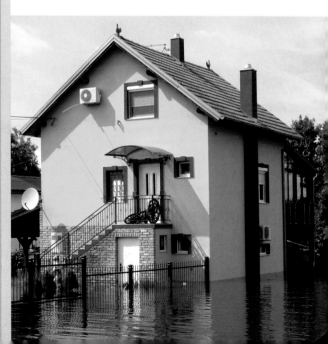

SCALE IT UP

Known as the Saffir–Simpson hurricane wind scale, this classification system is used to define the intensity and damage potential of sustained winds. First, tropical depressions and tropical storms develop before a hurricane is declared. Tropical depressions have a maximum sustained wind speed of 38 miles per hour (61 kph), while tropical storms have sustained wind speeds of 39–73 mph (63–117 kph).

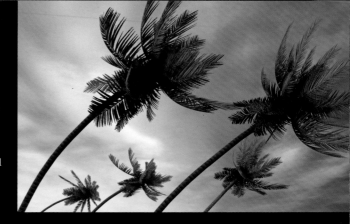

CATEGORY	SUSTAINED WIND SPEEDS	STORM SURGE HEIGHTS	POTENTIAL DAMAGE
1	74–95 mph (119–153 kph)	4–5 ft (1.2–1.5 m)	Some damage: Well-constructed homes could have damage to roof, shingles, vinyl siding, and gutters. Large branches of trees will snap; shallowly rooted trees may be toppled. Damage to power lines and poles may lead to power outages lasting several days.
2	96–110 mph (155–177 kph)	6–8 ft (1.8–2.4 m)	Extensive damage: Well-constructed homes may sustain major roof and siding damage. Shallow-rooted trees will be snapped or uprooted and block roads. Near-total power loss is expected with outages lasting from several days to weeks.
3	111–129 mph (179–208 kph)	9–12 ft (2.7–3.7 m)	Severe damage: Well-built homes may incur major damage or removal of roof decking and gable ends. Trees will be snapped or uprooted, blocking roads. Electricity and water may be unavailable for several days to weeks after the storm passes.
4	130–156 mph (209–251 kph)	13–18 ft (4–5.5 m)	Devastating damage: Well-built homes may sustain severe damage with loss of most of the roof structure and/or some exterior walls. Most trees will be snapped or uprooted and power poles downed. Fallen trees and power poles may isolate residential areas. Power outages may last weeks to possibly months. Most of the area will be uninhabitable for weeks or months.
5	≥ 157 mph (≥ 253 kph)	≥ 19 ft (≥ 5.8 m)	Catastrophic damage: A high percentage of homes will be destroyed, with total roof failure and wall collapse. Fallen trees and power poles will isolate residential areas. Power outages will last for weeks to possibly months. Most of the area will be uninhabitable for weeks or months.

249 PREPARE FOR THE TEMPEST

If you act well in advance of a hurricane, you can reduce the risk of damage to your home.

TRIM YOUR TREES Remove diseased or damaged limbs, and strategically remove branches so that wind can blow through.

INSTALL STORM SHUTTERS A set of permanent hurricane shutters provides the best protection for your windows and doors.

SECURE VALUABLES Consider getting a safety deposit box or buying a waterproof document safe for any valuable personal items and copies of important paperwork.

BUY EMERGENCY SUPPLIES When a hurricane threatens, supplies are quickly sold out at many stores. Be sure to get yours well in advance.

STRENGTHEN GARAGE DOORS Homes can be destroyed by winds through damaged garage doors. Reinforce or replace yours if you can.

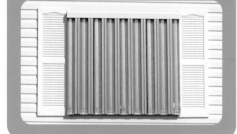

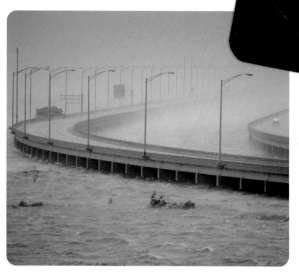

250 HANDLE A HURRICANE

When a hurricane watch is issued, it's time to prepare your home for a storm. Here are some of the things you should be doing.

First, prepare for evacuation: Fill up your gas tank, and pack all of your go bags and other supplies in your vehicle. Go over your evacuation plan, and consider leaving in advance of being ordered to do so. Prior to evacuating, turn off utilities and propane tanks as advised by local emergency officials.

Next, prepare your home: Secure your yard, as flying objects can damage your home or harm people. Protect windows with storm shutters or ½-inch (12mm) marine plywood covers. Shut all interior doors, and secure and brace external doors. Store drinking water; reserve more by filling clean bathtubs, sinks, and bottles.

If you live on a flood plain, be sure to take flood precautions as well. If you live in a mobile home, check your tie-downs and then evacuate as soon as possible.

251 BEWARE THE EYE OF THE STORM

The middle of each hurricane has a calm "eye" that can give the false impression that the storm is over. Often the worst part of the storm will happen after the eye passes over and the winds begin to blow from the opposite direction. Trees, buildings, and other objects damaged by the first part of the storm can be further damaged or destroyed by the second winds. Opposing winds begin suddenly, surprising and injuring unsuspecting people who left their shelter before they received an all-clear announcement from local emergency management officials.

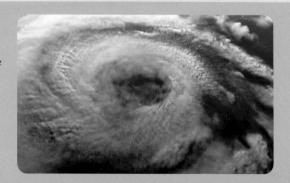

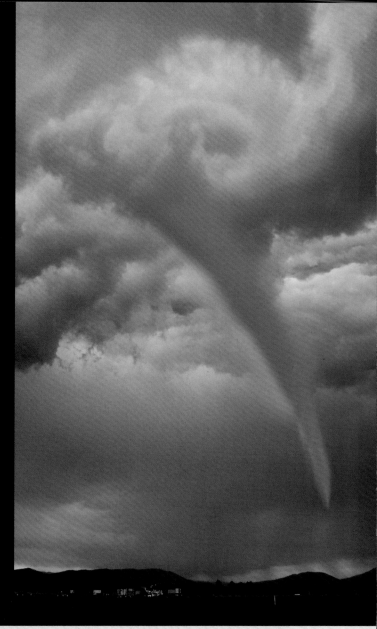

252
TELL WHEN A TWISTER IS COMING

Is that shape off in the horizon just an innocent cloud—or a deadly tornado? Here are some telltale signs to look for to know the difference.

SPOT A SUPERCELL A thunderhead with a hard-edged cauliflower look is called a supercell. This is a dangerous formation with interior winds of up to 170 miles per hour (274 kph).

WATCH FOR WALL CLOUDS These have clearly defined edges and look dense and, well, sort of like a wall.

GLIMPSE AT GREEN A sickly green hue in the sky can mean that a tornado is starting to take shape.

LOOK FOR LARGE HAIL Tornadoes will frequently emerge close to the hail-producing portions of a storm.

FIND A FUNNEL CLOUD A needlelike formation descending from a cloud's base indicates cyclonic activity. When a funnel cloud touches down, it becomes a tornado. Fortunately, most funnel clouds never touch down.

HEAR STRANGE SOUNDS Sounds similar to a train or a waterfall may be a sign of an approaching twister. If your ears pop, that means there has been a drop in air pressure, which is another danger sign.

253
JUDGE A TORNADO'S COURSE

If you're on the ground staring down a tornado, you can usually tell whether it's moving to your left or right. But if a tornado looks like it's standing still, it's hard to tell if it's heading toward you or away from you. If you're at all unsure, assume it's heading toward you and evacuate the area. Tornadoes often move southwest to northeast, so use a compass or a car's navigation system to avoid driving in the same direction. If you see a tornado, drive at a right angle to its path. Don't try driving directly away from the twister—that'll put you in the line of danger. There's an excellent chance that the tornado will overtake you, because twisters are fast and—sometimes downright impossible—to outrun.

254 STAY SAFE IN A TORNADO

A twister can touch down, and it's tough to know where you'll be or how bad the storm will get. Here's advice on staying safe in three likely situations, from a tornado that's hypothetical to one that's about to hit.

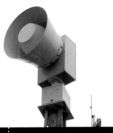

	HOME	CAR	OUTDOORS
TORNADO WATCH (POSSIBLE THREAT)	· Gather needed supplies. · Clear shelter of hazards. · Monitor broadcasts for pertinent details. · Watch local weather conditions for signs of supercell activities. · Check with friends and family members, and share plans and location information.	· Avoid back roads and unfamiliar places. · Head for home or a designated shelter. If weather becomes severe, pull over until conditions improve. · Avoid using hazard lights, which may distract other motorists. · Monitor broadcasts.	· If you're out camping, consider evacuating to a safer location. · Watch for tornadic signs in the southwestern sky. · Stash your gear inside your vehicle. · Contact a responsible person back home and fill him or her in on your situation and location.
TORNADO WARNING (IMMINENT THREAT)	· Stay away from your windows; do not open doors or windows. · Move to the basement or storm cellar if you have one, or to an interior room. · Get under a piece of sturdy furniture, such as a workbench or heavy table, and hold on to it. · If you're inside a mobile home, evacuate to a storm shelter or other sturdy building.	· Pull off the road and try to spot the tornado. · If you can see a funnel, determine its direction. · If you're in the tornado's path, drive immediately away at a right angle to its path. · If possible, seek shelter in a sturdy building or storm shelter.	· If possible, seek shelter inside the basement of a sturdy building. · Look for a low-lying area in which you can ride out the storm. · If you're in the tornado's path, move quickly to a ravine as far away from the twister's path as possible. · Stay low in order to avoid flying debris.
TORNADO DANGER (TOUCHDOWN)	· If you are not in your basement or a shelter, get into a bathtub or under a fixture that's been firmly attached to the floor. · Pull a mattress over yourself to protect yourself from any falling debris. · Lock arms with others. · Stay low and avoid the temptation to watch or film the tornado.	· Get out of the car. · Find a low-lying area, such as a ditch, and lie flat with your fingers locked together behind your head. · Do not go under an overpass; the risk of flying debris is much higher there. · If there's a boulder, put your hands behind your head and lie behind the side opposite the wind.	· Avoid the temptation to look up. Keep your head down on the ground. · Lie facedown with hands protecting your head in a low-lying area until the storm has passed. · Look for a sturdy object like a boulder, and put it between you and the twister.

255 PACK YOUR GO BAG

If you can prepare for an emergency in advance, you should. You never know when one will strike, and you never know how long it'll take to prepare on short notice. Here's what you should have packed and ready.

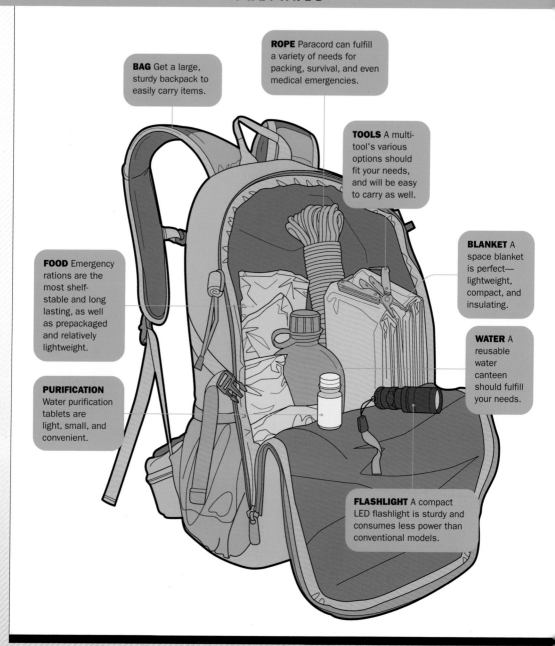

ROPE Paracord can fulfill a variety of needs for packing, survival, and even medical emergencies.

BAG Get a large, sturdy backpack to easily carry items.

TOOLS A multi-tool's various options should fit your needs, and will be easy to carry as well.

BLANKET A space blanket is perfect—lightweight, compact, and insulating.

FOOD Emergency rations are the most shelf-stable and long lasting, as well as prepackaged and relatively lightweight.

WATER A reusable water canteen should fulfill your needs.

PURIFICATION Water purification tablets are light, small, and convenient.

FLASHLIGHT A compact LED flashlight is sturdy and consumes less power than conventional models.

If you're caught off guard or can't get to your go bag, there's still hope. With a little luck and some rummaging around, you'll likely be able to put together an improvised go bag with the following suggested items to start.

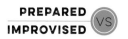

IMPROVISED

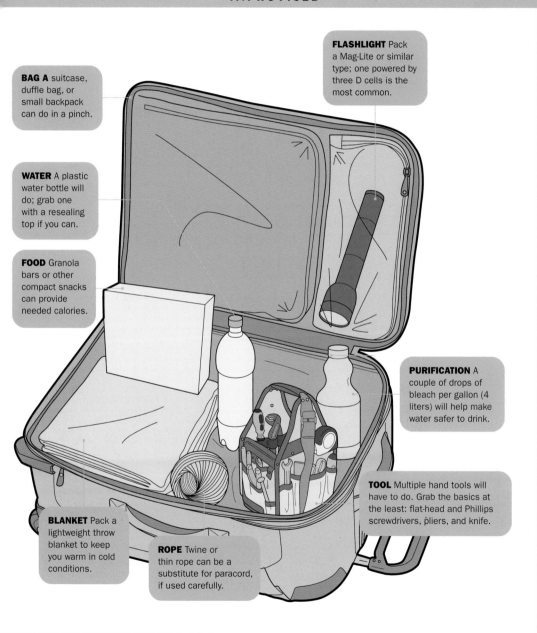

FLASHLIGHT Pack a Mag-Lite or similar type; one powered by three D cells is the most common.

BAG A suitcase, duffle bag, or small backpack can do in a pinch.

WATER A plastic water bottle will do; grab one with a resealing top if you can.

FOOD Granola bars or other compact snacks can provide needed calories.

PURIFICATION A couple of drops of bleach per gallon (4 liters) will help make water safer to drink.

TOOL Multiple hand tools will have to do. Grab the basics at the least: flat-head and Phillips screwdrivers, pliers, and knife.

BLANKET Pack a lightweight throw blanket to keep you warm in cold conditions.

ROPE Twine or thin rope can be a substitute for paracord, if used carefully.

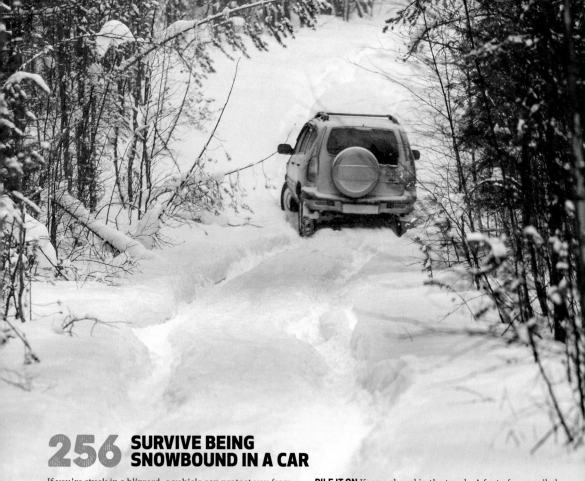

256 SURVIVE BEING SNOWBOUND IN A CAR

If you're stuck in a blizzard, a vehicle can protect you from wind and snow, and its visibility increases the odds that a search crew will find you. But in bitter cold, your car will likely feel like a freezer, because metal and glass offer no insulation. Thankfully snow offers remarkable insulation, which helps keep you warm inside your car.

STAY PUT Remain in your vehicle where rescuers are most likely to find you. Only leave if you see a better option for shelter, such as a building.

SIGNAL FOR HELP Check your mobile phone signal, and attempt to call, text, or post to social media that you've been stranded. If in a remote area, stomp large block letters in an open area spelling out HELP or SOS; line with rocks or tree limbs to be visible from the air.

GET NOTICED Tie a brightly colored piece of cloth to the antenna or top of the car. Check every few hours to make sure snow hasn't covered it. Keep snow off the car's hood so searchers can spot the color contrast from the air.

PILE IT ON Keep a shovel in the trunk. A foot of snow piled onto the passenger compartment will help turn it into a snow cave of sorts.

WARM UP Huddle with other passengers, make use of any clothing or blankets you have in your vehicle, and run the heater in short bursts to make the most of the fuel you have. Periodically clear snow from the exhaust pipe to prevent carbon monoxide poisoning. If you have candles, light one up—it'll deliver an amazing amount of warmth.

KEEP MOVING Exercise every so often inside the car to keep your circulation going.

RATION SUPPLIES Conserve food, water, fuel, and battery power. You never know how long you'll be stranded.

KEEP WATCH Take turns sleeping, as falling asleep can be deadly if it's cold enough. One person should be awake at all times to look for rescue crews and to keep an eye on the other occupants of the vehicle.

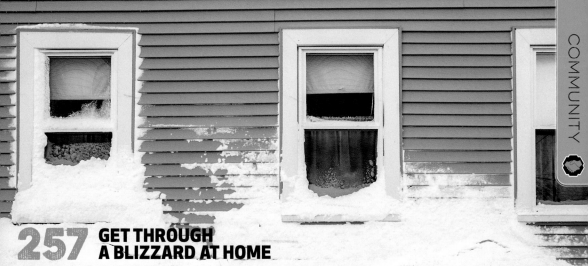

257 GET THROUGH A BLIZZARD AT HOME

Once a blizzard hits, it's best to stay in the protective shelter that your home provides. If you're in snow country, make a habit of checking the weather forecast daily; check your supplies and go shopping for extras if a storm is inbound.

STOCK UP Make sure your winter shelter-in-place survival kit is well loaded with the usual essentials, plus some extra blankets, sleeping bags, and heavy coats and other warm clothing. Stock up on sand, rock salt, and snow shovels to manage the snow after the storm is over. Consider buying some new board games or other forms of entertainment that don't rely on power.

WATCH YOUR WATER Severe cold can freeze pipes, leaving you without drinking water or the ability to use your bathroom. Store extra water in containers where it won't freeze.

WINTERIZE YOUR HOME Look for ways to make your home more resilient in the winter. Hang thick curtains over the windows for extra insulation. In the daytime, keep your curtains and blinds open to allow sunlight in to help warm your home. At night, keep them shut to trap heat inside.

STAY WARM Stock up on fuel for a wood-burning stove or fireplace. Huddle with others in a smaller interior room with no windows maximize warmth. Close doors to any rooms not in use to make better use of the available heat.

KEEP DRY If you must go outside, change out of wet clothing as soon as possible to prevent loss of body heat. Wet clothing loses its insulating properties, which can lead to frostbite or hypothermia (see item 110).

258 SET UP A SNOW PANTRY

If you loose power in a winter storm, one thing you don't have to worry about is keeping your perishables stored safely. All you need is a shovel, a footlocker, a cooler, or anything that is enclosed with a door to protect your food from scavengers.

STEP 1 Dig a hole in the snow or pile snow up and around the box to cover it in at least 1 foot (30 cm) of snow.

STEP 2 Place all perishable items into individual plastic bags to reduce odors that might attract animals.

STEP 3 Place food into the box and close it. Cover the opening with snow to further insulate your improvised freezer.

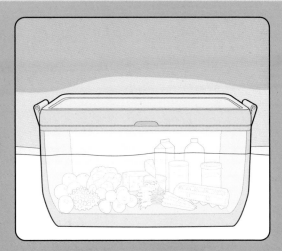

259 RIDE OUT AN EARTHQUAKE

When an earthquake strikes, the immediate priority is to get to a safe place to ride out the temblor, but where you are at the time will determine what you do next.

If you are indoors when the earthquake begins, drop to your hands and knees, and cover your head and neck with your arms. Move under any additional cover, such as under a sturdy desk or table, if you need to take shelter from the danger of falling objects. Stay away from glass, windows, outside doors and walls, or anything that could fall, such as items on shelves or furniture. Wait and remain inside until the shaking stops. Avoid doorways, as they do not provide protection from falling or flying objects.

If you are awakened by an earthquake, remain in bed and cover your head and neck with a pillow. Moving in the dark may result in more injuries than remaining in bed, as you won't be able to see debris or hazards, or judge how safe it is to move.

Should you be outdoors, get to open space if possible. Move away from buildings, streetlights, and utility wires. If you're in a dense urban area such as downtown in a city, you may be at less risk from falling debris if you get inside. Once you reach a safe spot, drop to your hands and knees and hold on until the quake stops.

If you're driving when an earthquake occurs, stop as quickly and safely as possible. Remain in the vehicle; avoid stopping near or under buildings, trees, overpasses, and utility wires. Proceed carefully once the earthquake has stopped, but be aware of aftershocks. Avoid underpasses, bridges, or ramps that the earthquake may have damaged.

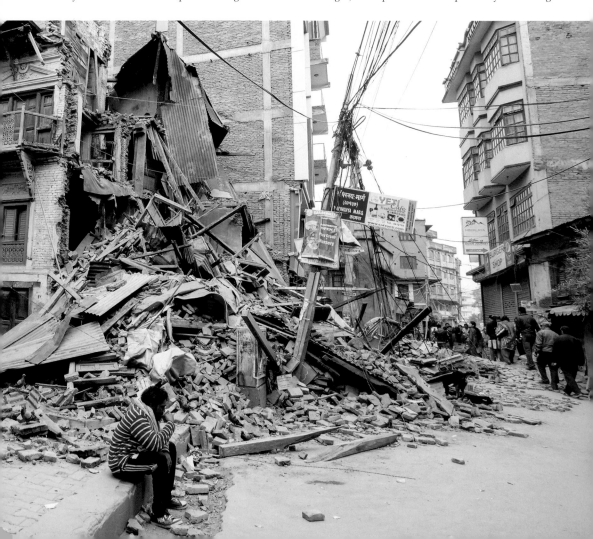

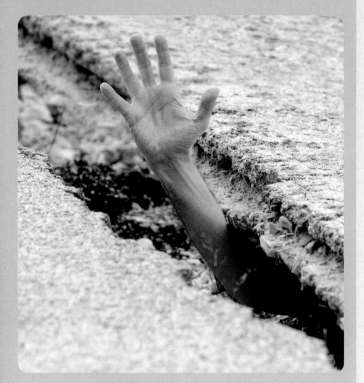

260 SURVIVE UNDER DEBRIS

The saying "earthquakes don't kill people, buildings do" reminds us of the risk of being trapped under debris or in a collapsed structure. If you survive an earthquake but end up trapped, you must be prepared to survive on your own with limited resources and space until rescuers can reach you. In order to improve your chances of survival, here are some important tips.

KEEP IN TOUCH If you have your phone, try calling, texting, or posting to social media. If none of those works, there may be an outage in the area. Turn your phone off to conserve the battery and try again every few hours.

DOUSE FLAMES Don't use a match or lighter to see where you are, as there could be a risk of explosion from gas leaks.

BREATHE EASY As dust settles from the collapse, cover your mouth and nose with a cloth. Avoid any movement that kicks up more dust, as that continues to make breathing more difficult.

SIGNAL FOR HELP You can call for help by tapping on a pipe or wall. If you have a whistle use it instead of your voice, as yelling will tire you quickly.

CONSERVE SUPPLIES If you have any food or drink on your person or accessible in the void, ration it carefully; you don't know how long you'll need it to last.

261 ASSESS A CONCUSSION

Concussions are common head injuries caused by a variety of circumstances, including car accidents, sports, a fall, or a blow to the head from falling debris.

Begin by checking to see if the victim has a bleeding head injury. If so, bandage the injury, but it's still common for concussions to develop localized swelling, or a "goose egg." Either way, visible external injuries are not a good gauge of severity, as even minor scalp wounds can have profuse bleeding. Instead, you should look for the following signs and symptoms:

- Balance problems or dizziness
- Confusion or brief loss of consciousness
- Drowsiness or feeling sluggish
- Double vision or blurred vision
- Headache
- Nausea or vomiting
- Sensitivity to light or noise

Have the person lie down and rest. Place a cold compress (frozen peas, cold pack, or ice, wrapped in a towel) on their head, and monitor them for the next 24 hours to ensure that they haven't gotten worse. Most symptoms of a concussion will resolve on their own, but if they persist or worsen, or if there are other serious signs, such as slurred speech, seizures, prolonged unconsciousness, or blood or clear fluid coming from their ears or nose, call for an ambulance and get medical help immediately.

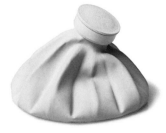

262 KNOW TSUNAMI WARNING SIGNS

A tsunami can move through deep water at more than 600 miles per hour (965 kph), crossing an ocean in less than a day. It won't slow in shallower waters; in fact, it speeds up. Go to high ground if you notice any one of these signs; don't wait for more than one sign or an official warning. Authorities may not have time to send an alert before the tsunami reaches land.

CHECK FOR QUAKES Earthquakes in a coastal region are a significant warning sign. If you're near the earthquake, seek high ground; if the tremor occurred elsewhere, monitor broadcasts for warnings.

LISTEN TO THE SEA Roaring sounds may precede the arrival of a tsunami.

WATCH THE WATERS As a tsunami approaches land, coastal waters recede, creating a drawback trough that exposes normally submerged areas. When this happens, you have just minutes before the wave hits.

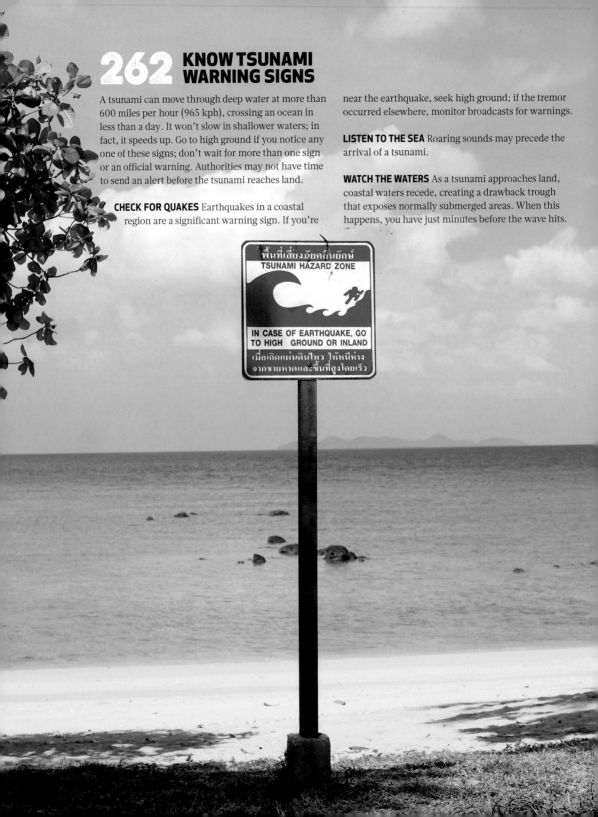

263 BRACE FOR IMPACT

Earthquakes aren't the only thing that cause tsunamis: volcanic activity, massive landslides, or large meteor impacts can all trigger one. Since the biggest tsunamis are as tall as 100 feet (30 m), you'll want to get at least that high above sea level to be safe. Anytime you're in a coastal area, think about where you would go in a big-wave emergency.

A tsunami is a series of waves, and the first may not be the most dangerous. A tsunami can last for several hours, and the wave series may come in surges that are anywhere from 5 minutes to an hour apart. Tsunamis can also travel up rivers and streams. During tsunami warnings, stay away from rivers and streams that lead to the ocean, and be sure to evacuate to higher ground even if you're up to 2 miles (3.2 km) away from the coast.

While in a coastal area, use your situational awareness to identify any escape routes to high ground. Plan on following designated tsunami evacuation routes (if they're established in your area) or simply heading inland and uphill as quickly as possible. Don't leave the safety of high ground until you are notified that the tsunami danger has past.

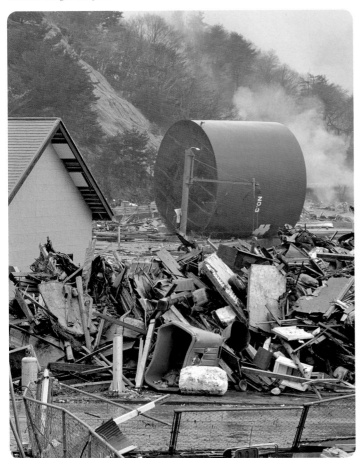

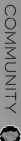

LIFE SAFETY APP
WEATHER

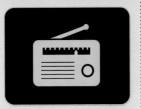

While having a weather radio is a great addition to your emergency kit, downloading a weather radio app is a great backup way for you to receive and access all of this information when you don't have the radio handy. There are many different apps available, including those that can provide small craft advisory along with other coastal warning features. Some apps are free and some charge for different features, including eliminating ads. There is no official mobile phone application available from the US National Oceanic and Atmospheric Administration (NOAA), but there are still many different apps to chose from which can stream and organize all the NOAA's weather information for you. The National Weather Service offers its own app-like interface which provides nationwide weather forecasts and information for your smartphone, and you can find other apps that deliver localized info and warnings for severe weather conditions in your area.

SUGGESTED APPS
- *NOAA Weather Radio*
- *NOAA Weather Radar*
- *Storm Weather Radar*
- *Stormshield*

Movies have typically portrayed red–hot lava as the biggest danger during an eruption, but there are really many more different types of potential hazards from volcanic activity, and lava is the least dangerous of them.

Molten rock usually flows relatively slowly, but lava is only the most commonly known part of an eruption. Along with lava, volcanoes will also eject other fallout—there are various pyroclastic materials, ranging in size from fragments to giant rocks, that can be thrown a short distance or ejected into the upper atmosphere. Volcanos also release hot gases that produce acid rain and air pollution that can spread far on wind currents, affecting regional or global climate.

In an eruption, water, debris, ash, and other materials can combine into a heavy slurry that can move quickly and with destructive force. The heat from the eruption can melt snowpack or divert rivers or streams, leading to flash floods. An erupting volcano can also trigger landslides, avalanches, earthquakes, and tsunamis.

After an eruption, seek a reliable source of emergency information to determine which hazards you may be facing, and respond accordingly. Prepare to evacuate; avoid areas downwind and river valleys downstream of the volcano.

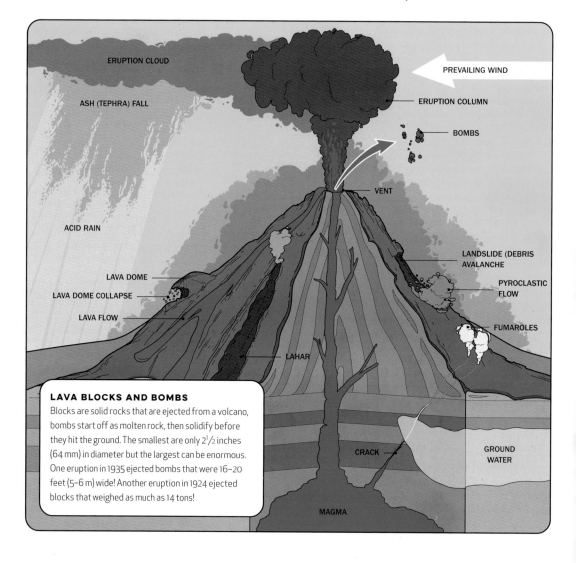

ERUPTION CLOUD

PREVAILING WIND

ASH (TEPHRA) FALL

ERUPTION COLUMN

BOMBS

VENT

ACID RAIN

LANDSLIDE (DEBRIS AVALANCHE)

LAVA DOME

LAVA DOME COLLAPSE

PYROCLASTIC FLOW

LAVA FLOW

FUMAROLES

LAHAR

CRACK

GROUND WATER

MAGMA

LAVA BLOCKS AND BOMBS

Blocks are solid rocks that are ejected from a volcano, bombs start off as molten rock, then solidify before they hit the ground. The smallest are only $2^1/2$ inches (64 mm) in diameter but the largest can be enormous. One eruption in 1935 ejected bombs that were 16–20 feet (5–6 m) wide! Another eruption in 1924 ejected blocks that weighed as much as 14 tons!

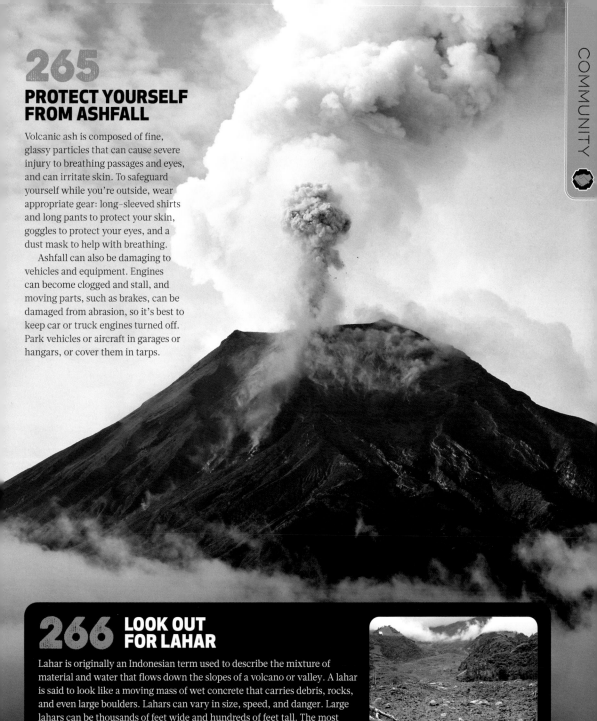

265
PROTECT YOURSELF FROM ASHFALL

Volcanic ash is composed of fine, glassy particles that can cause severe injury to breathing passages and eyes, and can irritate skin. To safeguard yourself while you're outside, wear appropriate gear: long-sleeved shirts and long pants to protect your skin, goggles to protect your eyes, and a dust mask to help with breathing.

Ashfall can also be damaging to vehicles and equipment. Engines can become clogged and stall, and moving parts, such as brakes, can be damaged from abrasion, so it's best to keep car or truck engines turned off. Park vehicles or aircraft in garages or hangars, or cover them in tarps.

266
LOOK OUT FOR LAHAR

Lahar is originally an Indonesian term used to describe the mixture of material and water that flows down the slopes of a volcano or valley. A lahar is said to look like a moving mass of wet concrete that carries debris, rocks, and even large boulders. Lahars can vary in size, speed, and danger. Large lahars can be thousands of feet wide and hundreds of feet tall. The most dangerous ones flow much faster than humans can run, up to 60 miles per hour (100 kph), and can flow for hundreds of miles before coming to rest.

267 HANDLE A HAZMAT EVENT

Hazmat, short for hazardous materials, is a broad term that can mean any number of dangerous solids, gases, or liquids, including substances that are radioactive, flammable, explosive, corrosive, oxidizing, biohazardous, toxic, or pathogenic. If you live or work near railway lines, freeways, or industrial complexes, you're at higher risk, as those areas are more likely to be the site of an incident.

STAY INFORMED Tune in to local radio or TV broadcasts or trusted internet news sources to stay up to date on the situation, and also make sure you're signed up for the emergency notification system for your area (see item 230). If you have been notified to evacuate, pack some bags in advance; if given no notice, grab your go bag. As you leave, keep all car windows shut, and set your air conditioner to recirculate air inside the car.

AVOID THE DANGER ZONE If you end up caught outdoors when the hazmat warning is issued, cover your face as completely as possible, and stay upwind, uphill, and upstream of the hazmat incident location, preferably at least 1 mile (1.6 km) away until you can find appropriate shelter.

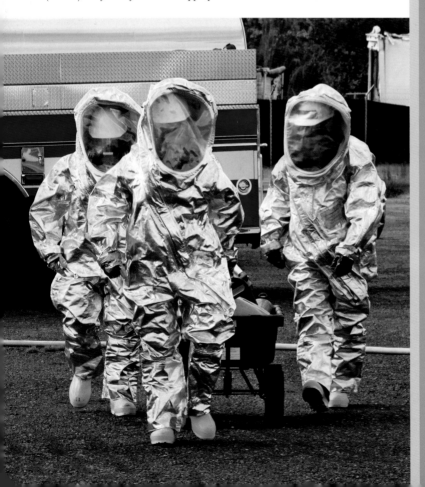

268 DECONTAMINATE YOURSELF

If you're unlucky enough to get any hazardous materials on your person, and there are no nearby emergency responders to help decontaminate you, it's time for you to take action yourself.

STEP 1 Strip off all your clothing immediately and seal it inside a plastic bag. Do not pull clothes off over your head; instead, use scissors to cut the clothing away. Also, while you are undressing, avoid touching your eyes, nose, or mouth, as you could introduce dangerous chemicals into your body by doing so.

STEP 2 If the hazardous material is in powder form and it is still visible, brush off as much as you can before getting into a shower. Scrub and rinse all affected areas for at least 15 minutes. Remove contact lenses and place them in the same bag as your clothes.

STEP 3 Put on fresh clothes and double-bag the contaminated clothing. Put the bags in a safe place, and do not handle them further until safe procedures to do so are advised by emergency response personnel.

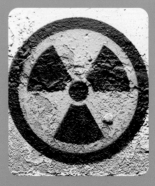

269 GET A DISASTER UNDER YOUR THUMB

If you spot a chemical spill, fire, or gas cloud, and you're not sure of the material being released, it's best to get far enough back to avoid getting contaminated by the hazmat incident. One easy trick is literally a rule of thumb.

Spot the incident site and extend your arm toward it. Line up your thumb with the site; if you can obscure the entire area with your thumb, then you're at a safe distance for the moment. If your thumb doesn't cover it, then continue moving away from the area until it does. Be sure to move upwind, uphill, and upstream from the incident if at all possible.

270 SEAL YOUR HOME

As soon as you are informed of a hazmat problem nearby, move indoors to limit exposure unless you're told to evacuate. In some cases the authorities may advise sealing your home. Here's how you can accomplish that.

STEP 1 Close any vents leading to the outside, including your fireplace damper. Turn off all of your air conditioners, fans, and ventilation systems.

STEP 2 Use plastic sheeting and duct tape to seal windows and doors. If you run out of plastic sheeting, you can improvise by using some aluminum foil, or even wax paper, to seal around air conditioner vents, kitchen and bathroom exhaust fans, and clothes dryer vents.

STEP 3 Close and lock exterior doors and windows so that no one can enter or leave after you seal the house.

STEP 4 Move to an aboveground room that has the least number of windows and doors. Once you're inside with all needed supplies, seal off any conduits leading into the room with duct tape, close all interior doors, and place towels at the bottom of doors to limit air circulation within the house.

271 STUDY SOLAR FLARES

A solar flare occurs when magnetic energy builds up in the sun's atmosphere and then suddenly released, thus emitting radiation across much of the electromagnetic spectrum. The amount of energy released can be massive—the equivalent of millions of thermonuclear bombs exploding simultaneously.

Flares are rated in various classes according to their intensity, similar to the Richter scale for earthquakes, in that each category is 10 times stronger than the one before it. A-, B-, and C-class flares have no significant impacts, but M-class eruptions can generate brief radio blackouts at the poles and cause minor radiation increases that can endanger orbiting astronauts. X-class flares, however, can potentially affect systems on a planet-wide scale, triggering a number of impacts on technology-dependent systems.

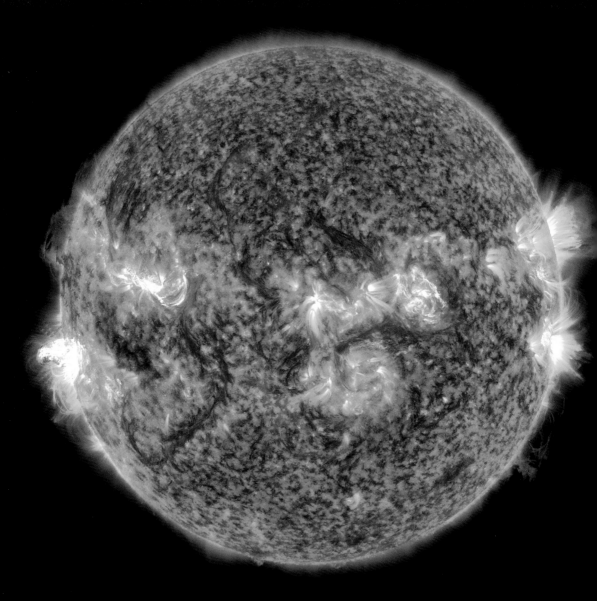

272 BE AWARE OF X-CLASS FLARES

The strongest class of solar flares can have a serious effect on technologically dependent systems, several of which can impact millions of people regionally or on large parts of the globe.

An X-class solar flare can disrupt GPS signals, thus hindering not only navigation critical to aviation, shipping, and personal use, but also global financial systems dependent on GPS signals to time-stamp transactions. Likewise, the flare can interrupt satellite-based TV, radio, Internet, and voice communications, such as satellite phones.

Electrical power grids can also suffer disruption from an X-class flare. While measures have been taken to prevent widespread problems, the distribution system may still be vulnerable.

Other impacts can include spacecraft anomalies as well as disruptions in telephone systems, public transportation systems, fuel distribution systems, pipelines and drilling, and air- and ship-based magnetic surveys.

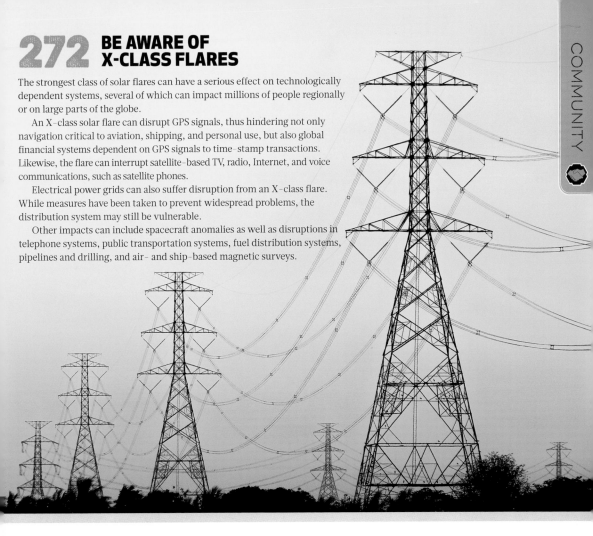

273 PREPARE FOR SPACE WEATHER

Your general disaster-planning efforts will also apply to space weather, but, obviously, there is really nothing preventative possible, given the cosmic nature of the threat. Being aware of the impacts and making plans to cope with them are the best way to handle this particular type of disaster.

The three types of effects you are likely to deal with are blackouts, electronics failures, and GPS or communications disruptions. To cope with a lack of navigation, paper maps in your car disaster kit will aid your ability to navigate not only during a solar flare but anytime your GPS isn't able to acquire a signal. Since communications will also likely be affected, having predesignated meeting places for members of your household allow you to convene even when you can't directly communicate.

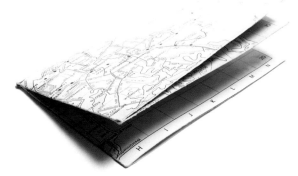

274 FORTIFY YOUR HOME

Preparing for emergencies and disasters doesn't mean just grabbing a go bag or packing a suitcase. If you need to shelter in place, your home could stand a bit of armoring and equipping too.

PREPARED

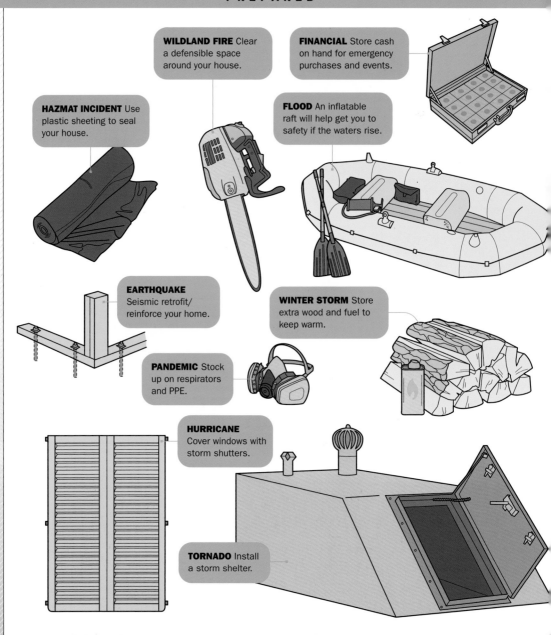

WILDLAND FIRE Clear a defensible space around your house.

FINANCIAL Store cash on hand for emergency purchases and events.

HAZMAT INCIDENT Use plastic sheeting to seal your house.

FLOOD An inflatable raft will help get you to safety if the waters rise.

EARTHQUAKE Seismic retrofit/ reinforce your home.

WINTER STORM Store extra wood and fuel to keep warm.

PANDEMIC Stock up on respirators and PPE.

HURRICANE Cover windows with storm shutters.

TORNADO Install a storm shelter.

If you're really pressed for time and haven't been able to prepare your house along with the rest of your possessions, there are still plenty of ways that you can make your home a safer shelter.

PREPARED VS **IMPROVISED**

IMPROVISED

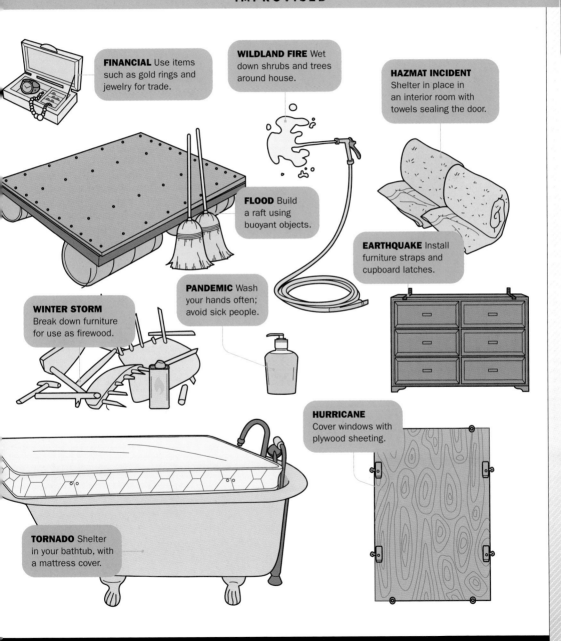

FINANCIAL Use items such as gold rings and jewelry for trade.

WILDLAND FIRE Wet down shrubs and trees around house.

HAZMAT INCIDENT Shelter in place in an interior room with towels sealing the door.

FLOOD Build a raft using buoyant objects.

EARTHQUAKE Install furniture straps and cupboard latches.

PANDEMIC Wash your hands often; avoid sick people.

WINTER STORM Break down furniture for use as firewood.

HURRICANE Cover windows with plywood sheeting.

TORNADO Shelter in your bathtub, with a mattress cover.

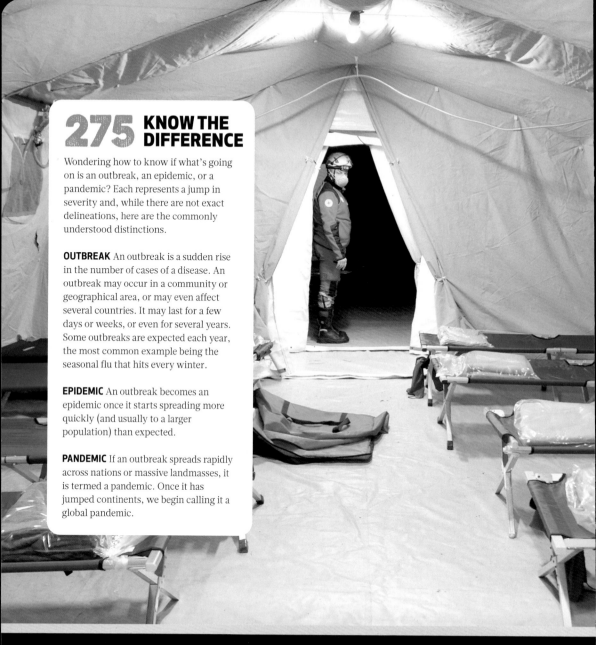

275 KNOW THE DIFFERENCE

Wondering how to know if what's going on is an outbreak, an epidemic, or a pandemic? Each represents a jump in severity and, while there are not exact delineations, here are the commonly understood distinctions.

OUTBREAK An outbreak is a sudden rise in the number of cases of a disease. An outbreak may occur in a community or geographical area, or may even affect several countries. It may last for a few days or weeks, or even for several years. Some outbreaks are expected each year, the most common example being the seasonal flu that hits every winter.

EPIDEMIC An outbreak becomes an epidemic once it starts spreading more quickly (and usually to a larger population) than expected.

PANDEMIC If an outbreak spreads rapidly across nations or massive landmasses, it is termed a pandemic. Once it has jumped continents, we begin calling it a global pandemic.

276 BE AWARE OF ARDS

People who end up in intensive care due to Covid-19 often suffer from acute respiratory distress syndrome, or ARDS, which impairs the lungs' ability to exchange oxygen and carbon dioxide. This can result in organ failure, brain damage, abnormal heart rhythms, and other serious conditions. The signs and symptoms of ARDS can begin within hours to days of infection; treatment uses a ventilator. Globally, ARDS affects more than 3 million people a year, as it can also occur from conditions such as pneumonia, sepsis, severe burns, and smoke inhalation. ARDS has a mortality rate of approximately 40% and even for those who survive, a decreased quality of life is sadly common.

277 USE BEST PRACTICES

While the specifics of any outbreak will keep changing and evolving as the virus does, there are some basic practices that are almost always appropriate.

☐ **WASH YOUR HANDS** If you're feel like you're washing your hands too often and for too long, you're probably doing it just enough.

☐ **USE HAND SANITIZER** If you can't wash your hands with soap and water, then this is the next best thing.

☐ **WEAR A MASK** A cloth or dust mask works fine to protect others from droplet transmission.

☐ **COVER YOUR MOUTH** Cough or sneeze into the crook of your arm if you don't have a tissue.

☐ **DON'T TOUCH YOUR FACE** Wearing a face mask helps keep your hands off your nose and mouth, but remember to not touch your eyes either, as an infection get into your system that way as well.

☐ **WEAR SAFETY GLASSES** To protect your eyes from airborne pathogens and keep you from touching your eyes.

☐ **KEEP AWAY** Consider 6 feet (2 m) as a minimum standard to avoid aerosol transmission from people nearby, even if they have no symptoms.

☐ **STAY HOME** Feeling sick? Stay home to avoid infecting others and seek medical attention if you feel worse.

☐ **PROTECT OTHERS** If someone in your household is sick, assume you also are contagious.

☐ **SHELTER IN PLACE** Remaining at home is the safest way to avoid exposure.

☐ **WIPE IT DOWN** Disinfect doorknobs, alarm keypads, or frequently touched surfaces, especially anything else you touch when first entering your home.

☐ **RINSE OFF** If you must go anywhere, change clothes and shower as soon as you get home.

☐ **PRACTICE SELF CARE** Eating well, sleeping well, and exercising regularly can bolster your immune system.

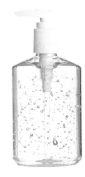

278 FOCUS ON CORONAVIRUS

Coronaviruses cause diseases in humans, mammals, and birds; when one crosses between species, it can go from being be mild in the original species to deadly in others. Often these start as a novel CoronaVirus (nCoV), the term for a medically significant new coronavirus . In humans the viruses cause respiratory tract infections which can range from mild to lethal. It is estimated about 15% of common colds in humans are caused by coronaviruses. In recent decades, several zoonotic coronaviruses (those that began with an animal strain and crossed over to us) have caused series outbreaks.

SARS The severe acute respiratory syndrome coronavirus (SARS-CoV) led to the 2002–2004 SARS outbreak. Over 8,000 people from 29 different countries and territories were infected, and at least 774 died worldwide with a fatality rate of 9.2%. SARS is known to have crossed over from to humans either directly from horseshoe bats or by way of wild civet meat sold at a local market in Guangdong, China.

MERS The first outbreak of Middle East respiratory syndrome-related coronavirus (MERS-CoV), was the 2012 MERS outbreak in the Middle East, followed by the 2015 MERS outbreak in South Korea and the 2018 MERS outbreak centered in Saudi Arabia. MERS has been genetically linked to Camels and Egyptian tomb bats as the zoonotic source of human infection. Globally MERS patients were reported in over 25 countries, with almost 2500 cases worldwide and over 850 deaths reported, giving it a fatality rate of 36%.

COVID-19 The Coronavirus 2 (SARS-CoV-2), the cause of the global COVID-19 pandemic, is a strain of the original SARS virus. The first known patient was infected in Wuhan, the capital of China's Hubei province, in November 2019. The virus subsequently spread to all provinces of China and to more than 150 other countries worldwide. Most people with COVID-19 recovered. For those who do not, the time from development of symptoms to death has been between 6 and 41 days, with an average 14 days. From a global perspective, the infection fatality rate is estimated to be up to 0.4%. However, of those who are admitted the hospital, the fatality rate is much higher, with a death to case ratio of approximately 6.2% at the time of writing.

279 UNDERSTAND THE TERMINOLOGY

With the news cycle being faster than ever, it's important to recognize that sometimes the media doesn't use scientific or medical terms correctly and that can cause confusion. To be well informed, you'll do well to know the basic terminology of pandemics.

CLUSTER A collection of cases occurring in the same place at the same time. If clusters are of sufficient size and severity, they may be upgraded to an outbreak.

COMMUNITY TRANSMISSION The term for cases of infection in persons who haven't traveled recently and have no connection to a known case. Also called "community spread."

CONTACT TRACING The practice of identifying and locating people who have been exposed to a known contagious person. They are then either asked to self-quarantine or brought in for observation in order to prevent transmission.

CONTAGIOUS Transmissible by direct or indirect contact with an infected person or thing. For example, the coronavirus is both contagious and infectious. Anything that is contagious is also infectious, but the reverse is not necessarily true.

DROPLET TRANSMISSION How a contagious disease is spread when it involves relatively large, short-range respiratory droplets produced by sneezing, coughing, or talking. Also called "aerosol transmission."

EPIDEMIC The rapid spread of disease to a large number of people across a very large area within a short period of time.

FLATTEN THE CURVE This refers to the goal of slowing a virus's spread to reduce the peak number of cases. This does not necessarily decrease the total number of cases; it just spreads them out over a longer period so that hospitals can cope with the number of patients at any given time rather than being overwhelmed.

HERD IMMUNITY A form of community protection from a disease that occurs when a large percentage has become immune, whether through previous infections or vaccination, thereby providing some measure of protection for individuals who are not yet immune.

INFECTIOUS Producing, capable of producing, or containing pathogens which can be transmitted. For example, food poisoning is infectious, but it is not contagious.

280 PACK EXTRA PANDEMIC SUPPLIES

Your emergency kits should already include these items, but if you're concerned about pandemics, or the news reports an increased risk, consider buying extra medical gloves, N95 respirators, and hand sanitizer. If the pandemic risk is very high, consider using disposable Tyvek jumpsuits and safety goggles as additional protection.

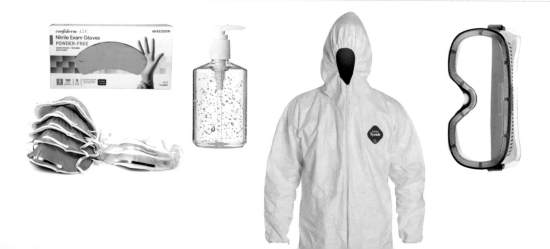

ISOLATION Methods used to separate patients infected with a communicable disease to isolate them from healthy persons, usually in a healthcare setting.

LOCKDOWN A government order preventing people from entering or leaving a specific area without special permission or performing essential functions.

OUTBREAK A sudden rise in the number of cases of a disease in a specific region.

PANDEMIC An epidemic that crosses international boundaries, affecting people on a multiple continents.

PPE This stands for "Personal Protective Equipment," the specialized clothing and equipment such as masks and hazmat suits used as a safeguard against physical, chemical, or biological hazards.

QUARANTINE Separating and restricting the movement of people exposed (or potentially exposed) to a contagious disease.

R0=X Pronounced "R-naught," an estimate of the average number of new cases of a disease that each infected person

generates. R0 estimates for the virus that causes COVID-19 are $R0 = \sim 2\text{-}3$, which is slightly higher than that for seasonal flu ($R0 = \sim 1.2\text{-}1.3$), but far lower than more contagious diseases such as measles ($R0 = \sim 12\text{-}18$).

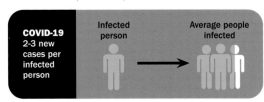

COVID-19 2-3 new cases per infected person

Infected person → Average people infected

SHELTER IN PLACE A directive issued by local, state or national government in which residents are either asked or ordered to remain at their place of residence, except to conduct essential activities.

SOCIAL DISTANCING Measures taken to reduce person-to-person contact in order to stop or slow down the spread of a contagious disease.

ZOONOSIS The process by which an infectious disease caused by a pathogen jumps from n animals to humans. More than two-thirds of human viruses are thought to be zoonotic.

281 BEWARE THE SUPER SPREADER

What is a "super spreader"? This is a person who infects a disproportionately high number of people, compared to number of people infected by the average sick person. In some of the cases of super-spreading, these infected people conform to the 20/80 rule. This means that roughly 20% of infected individuals cause up to 80% of the illness transmissions. A frightening proposition, if the disease is lethal. Perhaps the best known super spreader was Mary Mallon, also known as Typhoid Mary. Mallon was a cook for a number of different families in New York City. She was an asymptomatic carrier of typhoid fever, a potentially deadly disease caused by the bacteria *Salmonella typhi*. Mallon infected 51 people between 1902 to 1909. Three of those infected died from the illness. She was eventually placed under involuntarily quarantine (locked up) by public health authorities at Brothers Island in New York, until her death in 1938. If you don't have strong COVID-19 symptoms, but everyone around you gets sick after your close contact—you might be a super spreader. All the more reason for everyone to stay the hell at home.

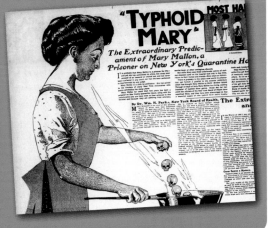

282 AVOID CONTAGIONS

Whether it's a pandemic or a seasonal flu outbreak, you can easily avoid infecting yourself or others.

Protect yourself by avoiding close contact with people who are sick. Regularly clean and disinfect surfaces or objects that you handle often, such as door handles or knobs, desktops, phones, faucets, and light switches. Avoid touching your eyes, nose, or mouth with your hands, since this is the most common way to contaminate yourself. Get plenty of sleep and exercise, manage your stress, stay hydrated, and eat a healthy diet.

In high-risk environments, wear a mask, and wash your hands or use hand sanitizer regularly.

Protect others by keeping your distance if you are ill. Stay home from work, school, and errands while sick. If you cough or sneeze, cover your nose and mouth with a tissue. (Alternatively, use your upper sleeve or elbow, not your hands.) If you have to be close to other people, again, put on a mask to protect others, and regularly clean your hands with soap and water or hand sanitizer.

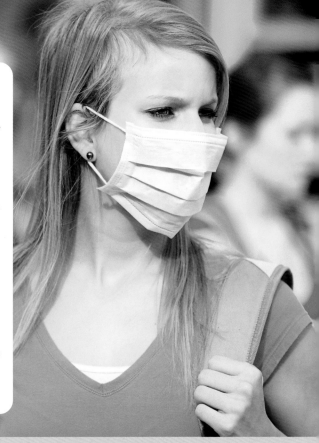

283 WASH UP

It turns out your mom was right: Washing your hands does make a big difference in preventing getting sick or infecting others. Surprisingly, studies found that even professionals in the medical field don't properly wash their hands, so take a moment to read how do it right.

STEP 1 Wet your hands with clean, running water (warm or cold), turn off the tap, and apply soap.

STEP 2 Rub hands together vigorously to scrub all surfaces, including the backs of your hands, between your fingers, and under your nails.

STEP 3 Continue for at least 20 seconds—it takes that long for the soap and scrubbing action to properly clean your hands. Want an easy way to time yourself? Imagine singing "Happy Birthday" twice.

STEP 4 Rinse your hands under running water.

STEP 5 Dry your hands by using a paper towel. Physically drying your hands helps remove bacteria.

STEP 6 If you are in a high-risk area, use your paper towel to turn off the faucet and open the bathroom door.

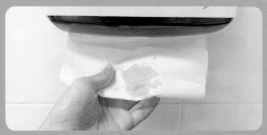

284 DON A MASK

Wearing an N95 mask can be a vital step in keeping yourself and others healthy. (That said, if you're not a medical professional, and live in one of the many areas where supplies are desperately short, do seriously consider donating your stash to a local hospital.

If you have the opportunity to isolate in your home, the donation could literally save a precious life. If you are an essential worker, or immune suppressed, or if your area is not experiencing shortages, a fresh, properly fitted N95 is definitely your best option.

Here's how to don it properly, for optimal safety, and how to remove it as well.

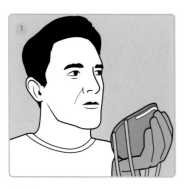

STEP 1 Always wash your hands thoroughly and then wear a fresh pair of gloves when handling safety equipment. Now, hold the mask in thepalm of your hand with the straps over your fingers and the mask's exterior facing the floor.

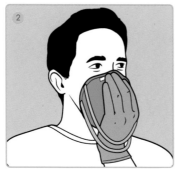

STEP 2 Place the mask onto your face, holding it so that it's fully covering your nose and mouth.

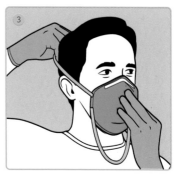

STEP 3 Pull the top strap up and over top of your head, and secure it behind your head, resting as snugly as possible above your ears.

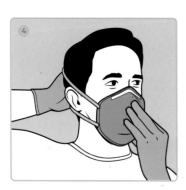

STEP 4 Take the lower strap and pull it over to place it behind your head and below your ears.

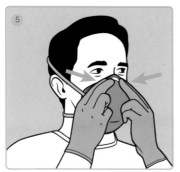

STEP 5 Mold the chevron-shaped metal nose piece of the respirator over the bridge of your nose to obtain a tight fit.

Finally, place your hands gently on the N95 mask and exhale. Adjust straps if the mask shifts during exhalation or if air escapes from the edges of the mask.

285 REMOVE IT RIGHT

Never touch the inside of mask, so as to avoid contaminating it. When removing a mask, always be sure to remove your gloves first so as to avoid contaminating it (after all, you're wearing your gloves to protect you, so just assume that they're contaminated by the time you need to remove the mask).

286 KNOW THE PLAN

Places where communities commonly gather, work, and play often develop their own emergency and disaster plans. If you or your family spend time at any of these facilities, especially as a student, employee, or volunteer, take the time to learn about what plans are in place. Some entities will provide this information on their website, but others may require attending meetings or inquiring directly. By informing yourself, you can better plan for how you or a member of your family might be affected by a disaster or an emergency based on where they might be at the time.

Consider looking into the disaster plans of places that you frequent, such as schools, workplaces, churches, day-care centers, and neighborhood associations, as well as stadiums, recreation areas, municipalities, and counties.

Additionally, if you live near one of these facilities, being informed about how their emergency response may affect you can help you plan ahead, and they may have additional resources available to you if they have been structured as a community disaster partner.

If you're not sure what to ask or look for in a plan, here are some good starting questions:

- What hazards, emergencies, or disasters are included?
- How are alerts and warnings issued?
- How often are plans updated, and is there a public review process to provide input?
- What are the local considerations for sheltering-in-place and evacuating?
- What else does the plan contain?
- Are plans available for download or review?
- Are there ways to learn more about preparedness?

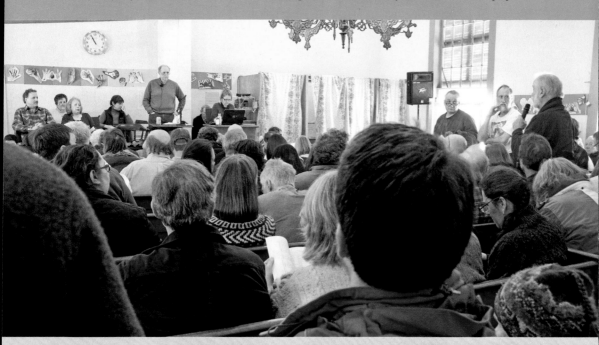

287 BE A COMMUNITY ACTIVIST

If there is no plan in an organization, consider appealing to its leadership to create a plan. Also, consider asking how to get involved in the planning process. Plans for disasters are best made when there is input and involvement from various stakeholders. If your initial efforts to set up a communal planning process fail, turn to other members of your local community and encourage them to voice their concerns. Last, you can contact politicians, local news media, or social media to raise awareness and concern. Since the goal is to create a resilient community, if you reach out to others, this is a good way to find common ground and build consensus and collaboration.

288 LEND A HELPING HAND

Volunteering is a great way to contribute to your community in a time of need, but it can also provide you the opportunity to learn some new skills, get access to training, and practice so that when you need to use those skills you'll be better prepared. Here are a few varieties of volunteer organizations and some of the skills you can learn from being involved.

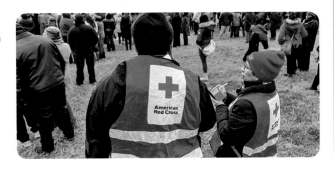

ORGANIZATION	LEARNING OPPORTUNITIES
AMATEUR RADIO EMERGENCY SERVICE (ARES)	HAM radio, emergency communications
CIVIL AIR PATROL (CAP)	Search and rescue, disaster relief
COMMUNITY EMERGENCY RESPONSE TEAM (CERT)	Light search and rescue, incident command, first aid, triage, fire safety, emergency response
NATIONAL WEATHER SERVICE (SKYWARN)	Storm spotting, severe weather assistance
RADIO AMATEUR CIVIL EMERGENCY SERVICE (RACES)	HAM radio, emergency communications
RED CROSS	Disaster response, first aid, shelter operations
SEARCH AND RESCUE (SAR)	Search and rescue, incident command

289 KEEP CASH ON HAND

When power is lost or telecommunications are down in your area, credit or debit cards will be useless. Checks might not be accepted either, leaving cash as the only way to buy supplies and food after a disaster. Here are some general guidelines to consider for where and how much to keep on hand. Carry the maximum amount you feel comfortable with and can afford. Also, by keeping amounts of cash in different places, it's unlikely that you'll lose all of your funds if you misplace one stash or get robbed.

WHERE	RANGE	THE BOTTOM LINE
PURSE OR WALLET	$20–100	Carry enough emergency funds to get you home safely.
EVERYDAY CARRY (EDC)	$20–100	This is the backup in case you accidently spend the emergency money in your wallet or purse.
CAR KIT	$60–100	Carry enough to fill up the tank at least once.
OFFICE KIT	$40–100	For when you're stranded at your office, keep enough to take a taxi or other transport home.
GO BAGS	$100	This stash goes toward general emergency funds for supplies.
HOME DISASTER SUPPLIES	$100/person	Secure enough for each person in your household to buy food, gas, and other critical post-disaster supplies.
RESERVE CASH	$200–2,000	Use when an extended disaster delays power and infrastructure for several weeks. Store enough for a month's worth of supplies.

290 SECURE YOUR CASH

One of the challenges in keeping cash at home is being able to hide it someplace where criminals won't find it easily. There is no perfect hiding place, but there are some options that are less prone to being easily found.

FREEZE IT Put the cash in a freezer bag, then wrap it up in tinfoil and label it "meatloaf" or something similar, as a fairly innocuous way to hide your valuables.

HIDE IN PLAIN SIGHT You can find safes resembling everyday items such as soda cans, deodorant, or cleaning products. They can't be locked, and don't hold very much, but they hide well out in the open.

KEEP IT SAFE A waterproof and fireproof safe is the best option if you want to properly secure your cash. Just be sure to anchor your safe so that it isn't easily carried off by potential thieves.

FAKE IT You can build or buy pre-made facades for wall switches, vents, drains, and other normal-looking home infrastructure in which to hide your valuables.

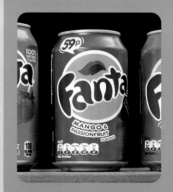

291 AUTOMATE YOUR CASH FLOW

Paying your bills can be a hassle even under conventional circumstances, but in a disaster it might be impossible. The same will go for trying to deposit a check from your employer. The postal service might not even deliver mail. All this means that important bills and hard-earned pay may not be getting taken care of. If your employer offers it, enroll in a direct deposit program to remove the hassle of lost checks. Also, consider using your bank's bill pay system to automatically handle all of your bills, including your mortgage, car payments, and credit card minimum payments so that, in an emergency, you won't also have to deal with worrying about your credit score.

292 PROTECT IMPORTANT DOCUMENTS

There are plenty of personal documents that, if they get lost, can cause problems and a lot of hassle to replace. It's helpful to keep electronic copies in cloud storage, but in the case of some important documents you'll need originals. Investing in a fireproof, waterproof document safe is an excellent way to protect those papers in the event of a disaster. Since you should keep your previous year's taxes in this collection, you can review and update all documents when you file your taxes. Here is list of recommended documents for you to review and consider.

IDENTITY	FINANCES
Driver's license · Other photo ID, including military · Birth certificate(s) · Social Security card(s) · Passport(s) and green card(s) · Naturalization documents · Child identity cards/dental records/DNA swabs	Financial accounts (checking, savings, CDs) · Home equity line of credit · Loans, including student and car · Credit card accounts · Retirement accounts (401k, IRA) · Investment accounts (stocks, bonds, mutual funds) · Previous year's tax returns (federal, state, and local)

FAMILY	HOME
Adoption papers · Child custody documents · Marriage license · Divorce license	Lease or rental agreement · Mortgage or real estate deeds of trust · Professional appraisals of personal property · Property tax statement

PETS	LEGAL
Proof of pet ownership and registration papers · Pet microchip information	Wills and trusts · Power(s) of attorney

INSURANCE POLICIES	HEALTH
Property/homeowner's/renter's insurance (including riders) · Auto insurance · Life insurance	Record of immunizations · Living will or Do Not Resuscitate orders

OTHER
Military discharge record (DD Form 214) · Vehicle registration and title

293 PLAN TO BE PREPARED

Various circumstances can lead you to a place where you are caught off guard and unprepared for the disaster at hand. You might be in an unfamiliar area or have to deal with an emergency you hadn't thought possible. Your plans may be overcome by new events and are now no longer current, or the support you had counted on is no longer available. Whatever happens, remain calm and use all your senses to stay safe and survive. Don't waste time and energy chastising yourself for what you should've done to better prepare. Stay focused and alert. Employing redundancy, being resilient, and having general survival priorities will improve your chances of getting through whatever sudden ordeal you might be facing.

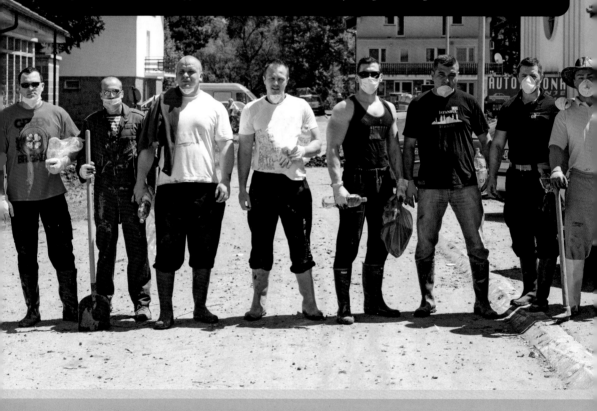

294 BACK UP YOUR PLANS

Regardless of whether you're creating emergency plans, stockpiling supplies, selecting equipment, or learning skills, you should have layers of redundancy just in case something fails. This means that when you're making plans, you should also design a plan B whenever reasonably possible. If there are other obvious options, consider coming up with multiple backup plans. It's impossible to plan for every contingency, but having several preplanned options can make the stress of an emergency easier to deal with, provided the plans are not so detailed as to burden you in the moment. You should also look at other resources in this way. Having multiple ways to treat water to make it safe to drink isn't just prudent; it may mean the difference between survival and tragedy. Skills should ideally not have a single point of failure either, so get yourself—and your loved ones—trained in first aid and other needed life-safety skills. In the end, as the famous Franz Kafka quote goes, it's "better to have, and not need, than to need, and not have."

295 BE RESILIENT

People with very few skills and almost no gear have survived seemingly insurmountable scenarios, simply because they had the right mindset to endure. These individuals tend to have some qualities in common that you can develop on your own. If you practiced them in lesser circumstances, they'll shine under the harsh light of adversity.

BE STRONG The strength of your will and the toughness of your mindset can trump physical prowess in survival situations. You must be willing to handle harsh conditions and suffering, and overcome personal weakness with a "do whatever it takes" attitude in order for you to prevail under the most extreme circumstances and events.

STAY MOTIVATED A common theme found in many survival stories is the survivor's devotion to a higher power or their intense desire to get back to family, friends, and loved ones. The ability to tap in to this kind of intense personal motivation is the mental aspect that keeps people going beyond all hope or reason.

LEARN TO ADAPT Adaptability and survival have always been closely related. The ability to adapt to changing events, challenges, and environments is one of the most impressive and necessary parts of a survivor's state of mind. It's tough to have to abandon a course of action, and it's very possible to fall into a fixed mindset or develop tunnel vision. If your approach isn't working, however, it's time to come up with a new way to handle the problem.

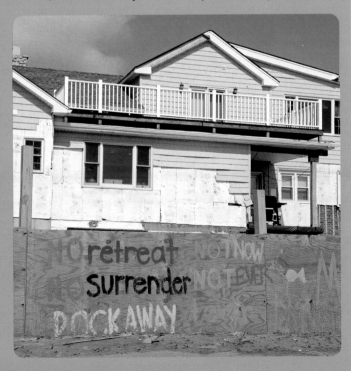

296 SET YOUR PRIORITIES

When you find yourself in a situation you are not prepared for, particularly when those circumstances appear especially dangerous, you'll need to focus on the right priorities in the right order to ensure your survival.

ADJUST YOUR ATTITUDE Remaining resilient is a chosen state of mind and necessary for survival.

GET FIRST AID Nothing else matters until a serious injury is treated or the victim is in the hands of a competent medical care provider.

TAKE SHELTER Protection from the elements is especially important in extreme weather conditions.

WARM UP Fire is critical for warmth, cooking, and signaling. Gather fuel and build a fire before darkness falls.

COMMUNICATE Try restoring electronic communications as well as making use of signaling devices such as mirrors, smoke, or marker dye.

FIND WATER A reliable water source is even more urgent when the weather is hot and dry.

FIND FOOD It is critical to be prepared by storing rations to see you and your family through a sustained emergency. If you run out, reaching out to friends and neighbors and may be your best option, or even foraging for edible plants, if you know what to look for.

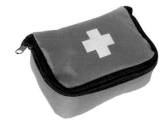

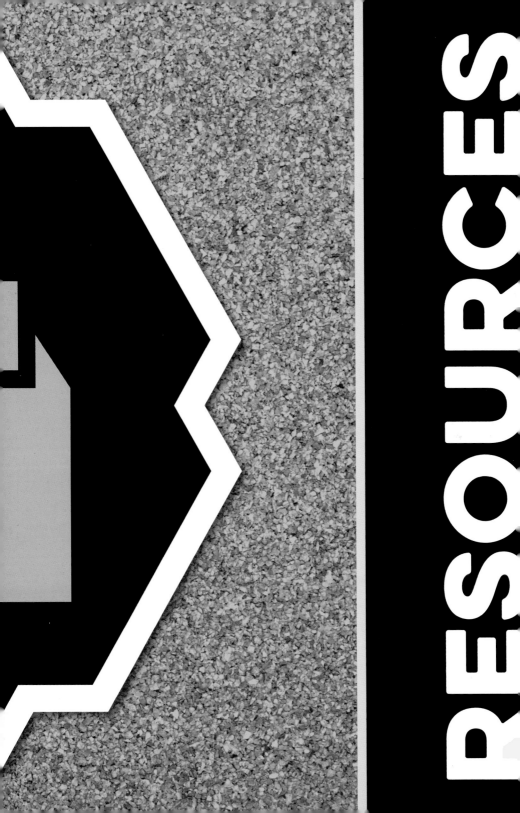

RESOURCES

297 COORDINATE AND EVACUATE

When disaster strikes, it's important to have a plan for where to go, whom to call, and how to meet up. This form makes it easy for everyone to know the details.

FAMILY CONTACTS LIST

OUTDOOR LIFE

FAMILY'S LAST NAME: _____

STREET ADDRESS: _____

CITY AND STATE: _____ **LAND LINE:** _____

EVERYONE WHO LIVES AT THIS ADDRESS

NAME: _____ **CELL PHONE:** _____ **SPECIAL NEEDS:** _____

EMAIL: _____ **WORK PHONE:** _____ _____

NAME: _____ **CELL PHONE:** _____ **SPECIAL NEEDS:** _____

EMAIL: _____ **WORK PHONE:** _____ _____

NAME: _____ **CELL PHONE:** _____ **SPECIAL NEEDS:** _____

EMAIL: _____ **WORK PHONE:** _____ _____

NAME: _____ **CELL PHONE:** _____ **SPECIAL NEEDS:** _____

EMAIL: _____ **WORK PHONE:** _____ _____

NAME: _____ **CELL PHONE:** _____ **SPECIAL NEEDS:** _____

EMAIL: _____ **WORK PHONE:** _____ _____

NAME: _____ **CELL PHONE:** _____ **SPECIAL NEEDS:** _____

EMAIL: _____ **WORK PHONE:** _____ _____

OUTDOOR LIFE

HOUSEHOLD EVACUATION PLAN

PETS

NAME: ____________ BREED: ____________ COLOR: ____________ MICROCHIP#: ____________

NAME: ____________ BREED: ____________ COLOR: ____________ MICROCHIP#: ____________

NAME: ____________ BREED: ____________ COLOR: ____________ MICROCHIP#: ____________

IF WE'RE SEPARATED DURING AN EMERGENCY, WHAT'S OUR MUSTER POINT NEAR HOME? ____________

IF WE CAN'T RETURN HOME, OR ARE TOLD TO EVACUATE, WHAT'S OUR MEETING POINT OUTSIDE THE NEIGHBORHOOD?

WHAT'S OUR ROUTE TO GET THERE? ____________

WHAT'S OUR ALTERNATIVE ROUTE IF THE FIRST ONE IS AFFECTED OR ELIMINATED BY DISASTER? ____________

IF FAMILY MEMBERS CAN'T REACH ONE ANOTHER, WHO'S OUR OUT-OF-AREA CONTACT PERSON?

NAME: ____________ ADDRESS: ____________

EMAIL: ____________ CELL/HOME/WORK PHONE: ____________

298 CHECK YOUR HOME FOR HAZARDS

Your home should be a safe haven, especially if you have kids. These simple checklists help you find and correct potentially deadly hazards.

OutdoorLife

CHEMICAL HAZARDS

☐ Be sure flammable liquids such as gasoline, cleaning products, and paint thinner are stored in a safe, well ventilated location, out of reach of children.

☐ Confirm that flammable liquids are stored well away from open flames, gas appliances, other possible heat sources.

☐ Verify that the storage containers have labels stating that they are approved by Underwriters Laboratory (UL) or Factory Mutual (FM).

☐ Make sure that all chemical storage containers have Mr. Yuk labels on them to warn children.

ELECTRICAL HAZARDS

☐ Examine extension and appliance cords to ensure that they are in good condition. Be sure they are not frayed or cracked, and have no loose prongs or plugs.

☐ Make sure that any extension cords currently in use are placed so as not to become a tripping hazard.

☐ Confirm that no extension cords are placed under rugs or over nails, heaters, or pipes.

☐ Ensure that all wiring is properly covered.

☐ Monitor all appliances to ensure that they operate safely and do not overheat, short out, smoke, or spark.

FIRE HAZARDS

☐ Keep old rags, papers, mattresses, broken furniture, clothes, curtains, and the like away from electrical equipment, gas appliances, or other possible sources of heat or flame.

☐ Keep fully charged fire extinguishers on each floor and ensure that they are serviced or replaced as needed.

☐ Safely dispose of all garden waste and dried grass clippings, tree trimmings, or pulled weeds.

☐ Replace the batteries in all smoke and carbon monoxide detectors annually.

FLOOD HAZARDS

☐ Check gutters and downspouts to be sure they are not clogged with debris.

☐ Inspect storm drains near your property. If they are clogged, contact your local authorities for follow-up.

☐ Inspect your property for possible flood risks. Consider storing sandbags and supplies for seasonal flooding.

ORGANIC HAZARDS

☐ Check if any of your houseplants are poisonous or toxic. If so, make sure they are out of reach of pets and children.

☐ Confirm there is no mold on the walls or ceiling of your bathrooms, kitchen, basement, or other rooms.

STRUCTURAL HAZARDS

☐ Consider securing water heaters, large appliances, bookcases, other tall and heavy furniture, shelves, mirrors, pictures, and overhead light fixtures by anchoring to wall studs.

☐ Consider moving heavy pictures or mirrors away from where people sleep.

☐ Move large or heavy objects to lower shelves.

☐ If needed, install flexible gas supply lines for the water heater or other gas appliances.

☐ Evaluate cabinet doors to see if any require latches or locks to keep items from falling out.

☐ Ensure lighting is appropriate for all areas inside and outside the home, especially stairs.

☐ Clear any clutter from hallways and stairways.

☐ Inspect and repair any cracks in the foundation or other parts of your home.

CHILD SAFETY MEASURES

☐ Install safety gates at the tops and bottoms of stairways; verify that they are securely mounted.

☐ Install guards around fireplaces, radiators, hot pipes, or wood-burning stoves; verify that they are securely mounted.

☐ Consider installing corner guards on furniture and other protection from sharp edges in the home as needed.

☐ Keep curtain cords and shade pulls out of reach.

☐ Set your hot water heater to a safe temperature of 120 °F (49 °C) or less.

☐ Store all prescription drugs and over-the-counter medicines in childproof containers and out of reach.

☐ Keep shampoos and cosmetics out of reach.

☐ Keep all sharp objects in the bathroom, kitchen, and other areas out of reach.

☐ Ensure that toilet seats and lids are left down when not in use.

☐ Keep all electrical outlets covered.

☐ Inspect beds or cribs to ensure they are mounted away from radiators or other hot surfaces.

☐ Verify that mattresses fit the sides of cribs snugly, and that crib slats are no more than $2^{3}/8$ inches (6 cm) apart.

☐ Confirm that toy boxes have secure lids and safe-closing hinges.

299 KNOW WHAT'S SAFE TO EAT

After a power outage, you may be torn between not wanting to waste valuable food, and the fear of food poisoning. Use these guidelines to keep you healthy.

FOOD IN REFRIGERATOR

HELD ABOVE 40 °F (4 °C) FOR MORE THAN 2 HOURS

Meat, poultry, or seafood (raw, leftover, or thawing; also includes soy meat substitutes, salads, lunch meats, pizza, cans that have been opened, and sauces with fish or meat)	**DISCARD**
Any soft, shredded, or low-fat cheeses	**DISCARD**
Hard cheeses such as cheddar, colby, swiss, parmesan, provolone, romano, or hard cheeses grated in can or jar	**SAFE**
Milk, cream, sour cream, buttermilk, evaporated milk, yogurt, eggnog, soy milk, or opened baby formula	**DISCARD**
Butter, margarine	**SAFE**
All eggs and egg-based products, such as puddings	**DISCARD**
Fresh fruits, if cut up	**DISCARD**
Pre-cut, pre-washed, and/or cooked vegetables, tofu, opened vegetable juice, garlic in oil, or potato salad	**DISCARD**

Opened fruit juices or canned fruits, along with fresh fruits, coconut, dried or candied fruits, and dates	**SAFE**
Vegetable or cream-based sauces, jam, opened mayonnaise, tartar sauce, and horseradish	**DISCARD***
	* if above 50 °F (10 °C) for over 8 hours
Soy, barbecue, and taco sauce, peanut butter, jelly, relish, mustard, catsup, olives, pickles, and vinegar-based dressings	**SAFE**
Opened creamy-base dressings or spaghetti sauce	**DISCARD**
Bread, rolls, cakes, cookies, muffins, quick breads, tortillas, waffles, pancakes, bagels, fruit pies, pastries, grains	**SAFE**
Unbaked dough, cooked pasta, rice, potatoes, pasta salads, fresh pasta, cheesecake, or cream-filled pastries or pies	**DISCARD**
Fresh raw vegetables, mushrooms, herbs, and spices	**SAFE**
Casseroles, soups, and stews	**DISCARD**

FOOD TYPE	STILL CONTAINS ICE CRYSTALS AND FEELS AS COLD AS IF REFRIGERATED	THAWED; HELD ABOVE 40 °F (4 °C) FOR MORE THAN 2 HOURS
Meat, poultry, and seafood	**REFREEZE** (Seafood loses some texture and flavor)	**DISCARD**
Milk and soft or semi-soft cheese	**REFREEZE** (Products may lose some texture)	**DISCARD**
Eggs (out of shell) and egg products	**REFREEZE**	**DISCARD**
Ice cream or frozen yogurt	**DISCARD**	**DISCARD**
Hard and shredded cheeses, casseroles with dairy products, cheesecake	**REFREEZE**	**DISCARD**
Fruits (juices and packaged fruits)	**REFREEZE** (Fruit's texture and flavor will change)	**DISCARD**
Vegetables (juices and packaged vegetables)	**REFREEZE** (Vegetables may lose texture and flavor)	**DISCARD** (If above 40 °F (4 °C) for more than 6 hours)
Breads and pastries (breads, rolls, muffins, and cakes without custard fillings)	**REFREEZE**	**REFREEZE**
Cakes, pies, and pastries with custard or cheese fillings	**REFREEZE**	**DISCARD**
Pie crusts, commercial and homemade bread dough	**REFREEZE** (Some quality loss may occur)	**REFREEZE** (Quality loss will be considerable.)
Casseroles (pasta and rice-based)	**REFREEZE**	**DISCARD**
Flour, cornmeal, nuts, waffles, pancakes, bagels	**REFREEZE**	**REFREEZE**
Frozen meals	**REFREEZE**	**DISCARD**

300 COMMUTE WITH A CONTINGENCY PLAN

If you're caught on your way to or from work when disaster strikes, having a range of options already planned means you're well ahead of the rest of the crowd.

OUTDOORLIFE

PUBLIC TRANSPORTATION OPTIONS TO AND FROM WORK

MODE	LINE	STOP	FARE

DRIVING OR BIKE ROUTES TO AND FROM WORK

	PRIMARY ROUTE	ALTERNATIVE ROUTE #1	ALTERNATIVE ROUTE #2
TO			
FROM			

OTHER TRANSPORTATION OPTIONS

	PHONE NUMBER	WEB ADDRESS	NOTES
TAXI			
COMMUTER BUS			
COMMUTER RAIL			
OTHER			

OUTDOORLIFE

COWORKERS WHO LIVE NEARBY FOR RIDE-SHARING

NAME	OFFICE	PHONE	MOBILE	EMAIL

CAR RENTALS NEAR WORK

COMPANY	ADDRESS	PHONE	WEB ADDRESS

HOTELS NEAR WORK

NAME	ADDRESS	PHONE	WEB ADDRESS

LOCAL TRAFFIC AND TRANSPORTATION INFORMATION

NAME	WEB ADDRESS	NOTES

LOCAL RED CROSS

ADDRESS	PHONE	WEB ADDRESS

301 RETURN TO A SAFE HOME

Once the crisis is over, you may well be facing a whole new set of challenges as you cope with the aftermath of a major natural or man-made disaster.

POST-DISASTER HOME ASSESSMENT CHECKLIST

OUTDOOR LIFE

BEFORE RETURNING TO YOUR HOME

☐ Find out if it is safe to enter your community or neighborhood. Follow the advice of your local authorities.

☐ Create backup communication plans with family and friends in case you are unable to call.

☐ If possible, leave children and pets with a relative or friend while you make your initial inspection.

☐ Bring food and water and pack protective clothing and boots.

DO NOT ENTER IF

☐ You smell gas.

☐ Floodwaters remain around the building.

☐ Your home was seriously damaged by fire or other natural disaster and the authorities have not declared it safe.

☐ You have any doubts about safety. Have your home inspected by a qualified building inspector or structural engineer before entering.

ASSESS THE EXTERIOR OF YOUR HOME, DOCUMENTING AND PHOTOGRAPHING ANY OF THE FOLLOWING

☐ Loose or damaged power lines.

☐ Broken or leaking gas and water pipes.

☐ Wild animals.

☐ Any instability; the building needs to be securely on its foundation.

☐ Cracks in your home's foundation or chimney.

☐ Damaged walls.

☐ Any collapsed areas on the roof.

☐ Broken windows or doors.

ASSESS YOUR HOME'S INTERIOR

☐ Beware of rodents, snakes, insects, or other animals that may be inside your home.

☐ If your home was flooded, assume it is contaminated with mold.

☐ Check the ceiling and floor for signs of sagging. The floor may be unsafe if it is wet or damaged.

☐ Check the sewage disposal system.

☐ Open doors and windows. Let the house air out before staying inside for any length of time if the house was closed for more than 48 hours.

☐ Open cabinets carefully. Be alert for objects that may fall.

☐ Take pictures of damage for insurance purposes.

☐ Keep records of the amount of time taken to remove debris and clean.

From *The Ultimate Emergency Survival Manual* (c) 2015. Download additional forms at www.josephpred.com.

OUTDOORLIFE

ASSESS YOUR HOME'S UTILITIES

☐ Even if you shut off all of your utilities before evacuating, perform your inspection as though they were on and posing a potential hazard. Because thy might be.

☐ Do not smoke while assessing your home.

☐ When re-entering the building, use a flashlight in case of a gas leak. Turn it on outside before entering, as it could produce a spark that can ignite leaking gas, if present.

☐ Smell for gas. If you smell natural gas or propane, or hear a hissing noise, leave immediately and contact the fire department. Once outside, turn off the gas supply, if you can do so safely.

☐ Check pilot lights to confirm whether they are lit or out.

☐ Call the gas or propane company before you turn the gas back on.

☐ Inspect the interior for any damage to electrical, gas, or water lines.

☐ Have a professional check your heating system before use.

☐ Look for sparks, or broken or frayed wiring.

☐ If the main power and water systems are on, turn them off until you or a professional can ensure that they are safe.

☐ If there is standing water in your home, do not enter your basement or turn the power on or off. Never use any electrical tool or appliances while standing in water. Do not use any electricity until a licensed electrician has inspected your home.

☐ If any appliances were touched by floodwaters, unplug them and have them checked by a qualified service person before operating them.

☐ If pipes appear damaged, turn off the main water valve.

☐ Have your tap water tested by authorities before drinking.

☐ Do not flush toilets until you know that sewage lines are intact.

ORGANIZE AND CLEAN

☐ Wear protective clothing, including N95 masks, gloves, and boots.

☐ Discard all perishable or frozen food that has expired or stored without proper refrigeration. When in doubt, throw it out.

☐ Sort contents to be repaired or discarded.

☐ Remove minor debris such as branches and trash.

☐ If you hire cleanup or repair contractors, verify that they are qualified and insured to do the job. Be wary of people who drive through neighborhoods offering help in cleaning up or repairing your home. Check references.

INDEX

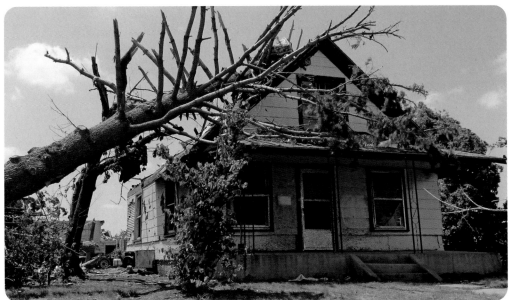

INDEX

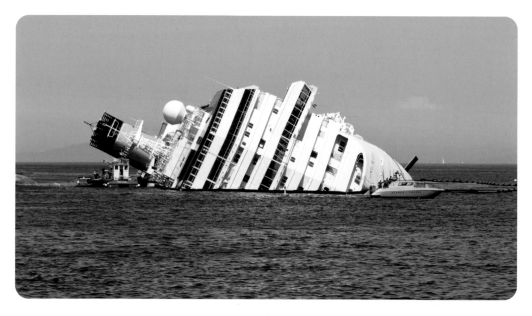

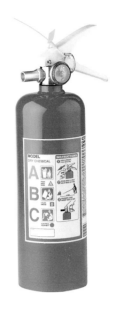

INDEX

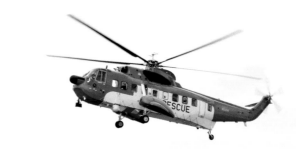

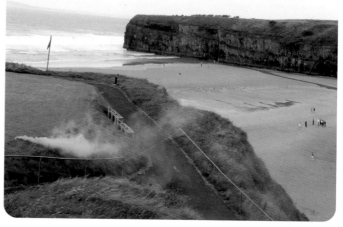

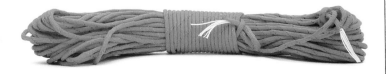

INDEX

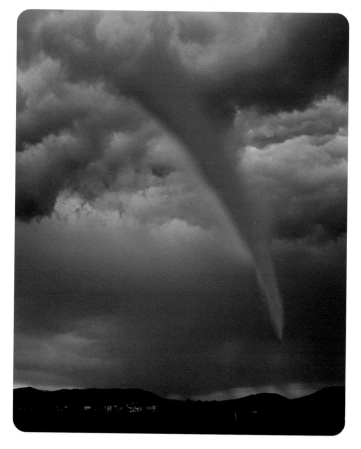

ABOUT THE AUTHOR

Joseph Pred has made a career in emergency and risk management, with over 20 years of experience in public safety, with a renaissance style background in emergency medical services, law enforcement, fire safety, emergency communications, incident management, mental health, leadership, safety, and risk.

Joseph's previous works include the *Outdoor Life* book *Show Me How to Survive,* and he regularly speaks at conferences on matters of public safety, risk, and temporary mass gatherings.

Currently he serves as CEO of Mutual Aid Response Services and Mutual Aid Safety & Risk. Learn more at www.josephpred.com.

ABOUT THE MAGAZINE

Since it was founded in 1898, *Outdoor Life* magazine has provided survival tips, wilderness skills, gear reports, and other essential information for hands-on outdoor enthusiasts. Each issue delivers the best advice in sportsmanship as well as thrilling true-life tales, detailed gear reviews, insider hunting, shooting, and fishing hints, and much more to nearly 1 million readers. Its survival-themed Web site also covers disaster preparedness and the skills you need to thrive anywhere from the backcountry to the urban jungles.

ACKNOWLEDGMENTS

I am grateful for the opportunity to share my knowledge and experience with you for this book, but I wouldn't have been able to do so without the immeasurable help of the colleagues, teachers, and mentors throughout the twenty- plus years of my career that have supported my professional development. It's impossible for me to name them all, but you know who you are.

I especially want to thank my friends and colleagues Barbara Denman, JohnRey Hassan, Humphrey Ogg, and Nicole Nasser for lending some of their expertise on some of the content for this book.

I also want to offer a special thank you to Amy, whose endless support throughout the entire writing process made it all possible.

Lastly, none of this would be possible without the guidance, support, and experience of my senior editor Mariah Bear. My sincerest thanks and gratitude for all the time and effort Mariah, and the entire team at Weldon Owen publishing who made this book possible, especially the efforts of Ian Cannon, Allister Fein, and William Mack.

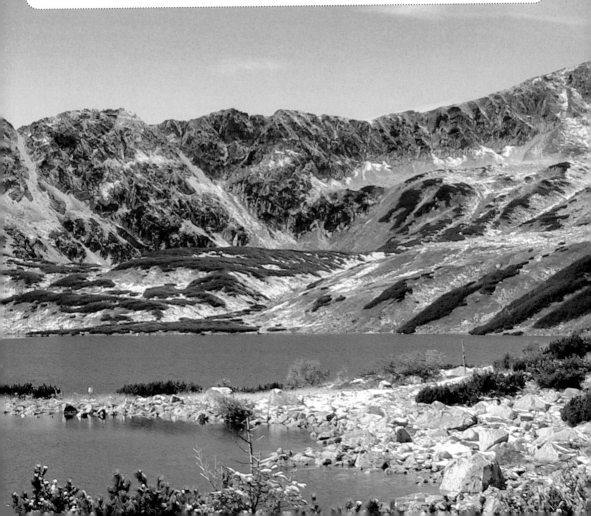

weldon**owen**

PUBLISHER Roger Shaw
ASSOCIATE PUBLISHER Mariah Bear
PROJECT EDITOR Ian Cannon
CREATIVE DIRECTOR Chrissy Kwansick
ART DIRECTOR Allister Fein
ILLUSTRATION COORDINATOR Conor Buckley

Weldon Owen would like to thank
Marisa Solís and Jan Hughes for editorial
assistance and Kevin Broccoli for
the index.

© 2020 Weldon Owen International
1150 Brickyard Cove Road
Richmond, CA 94801
www.weldonowen.com

ISBN 978-1-68188-531-5
10 9 8 7 6 5 4 3
2021 2022 2023 2024
Printed in China

OUTDOORLIFE

2 Park Avenue
New York, NY 10016
www.outdoorlife.com

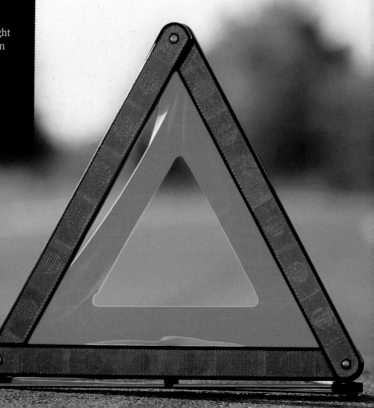